Psychosocial issues in palliative care

Edited by

Mari Lloyd-Williams

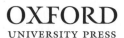

UNIVERSITY PRESS

Great Clarendon Street, Oxford OX2 6DP

Oxford University Press is a department of the University of Oxford.
It furthers the University's objective of excellence in research, scholarship,
and education by publishing worldwide in

Oxford   New York

Auckland   Bangkok   Buenos Aires   Cape Town   Chennai
Dar es Salaam   Delhi   Hong Kong   Istanbul   Karachi   Kolkata
Kuala Lumpur   Madrid   Melbourne   Mexico City   Mumbai   Nairobi
São Paulo   Shanghai   Taipei   Tokyo   Toronto

Oxford is a registered trade mark of Oxford University Press
in the UK and in certain other countries

Published in the United States
by Oxford University Press Inc., New York

© Oxford University Press 2003

A catalogue record for this title is available from the British Library

Library of Congress Cataloging in Publication Data
(Data available)

ISBN 0 19 851540 5

10 9 8 7 6 5 4 3 2 1

Typeset by Cepha Imaging Private Ltd., Bangalore.
Printed in Great Britain
on acid-free paper by T. J. International Ltd, Padstow, Cornwall

Dedication
This book is dedicated to my parents; and to Aled, Emily, Henry, Oliver,
Amy, and Sophie, who contribute so much joy.

Foreword

Professor Baroness Ilora Finlay of
Llandaff FRCGP, FRCP

When patients are terminally ill, providing psychosocial care for them and their families is complex. An interdisciplinary approach is essential if the complex, and often competing, needs of the patient and the different family members are to be met. In this book these problems are explored in depth to provide an evidence-based practical guide for the individual professional in the clinical team.

This book addresses the complex area of psychosocial care. It can be easy to think that by being nice and warm to patients, their needs will be in large part met. Needs assessment can be difficult, yet is being increasingly required by the commissioning services. The different screening tools for psychosocial distress are outlined here and have a particular role for teams where the care of the patient and family involves many different professionals. Knowing the right screening tool is important in care; all those teaching students in any of the healthcare disciplines need to know what could or should be done to detect distress and thereby help students to be more aware of the needs of patients.

One major casualty of the current team structures has been the continuity of care of patients when care becomes complicated. So the team issues around team approaches to the depressed or distressed patient are vital philosophical inputs which determine team behaviours and the experience of those on the receiving end of care. There are very real cultural issues in society today that require in-depth understanding. There are techniques to be learnt to help communication with those who have communication difficulties. Social and financial affairs are becoming increasingly complex in today's society—the terminally ill patient does not have time to wait for bureaucracy or for form filling.

Improving the quality of life of patients and their families takes an effort of urgency. It requires the carers to give of themselves and of their time and to have accurate expert knowledge as well as communication skills and competencies. It can be arrogant to believe that one professional can know all and that care is always as good as we intend it to be. Auditing care becomes vital in the quest to maintain high standards.

Many patients and their families are desperate to try anything that will improve their quality of life. They are keen to try complementary therapies yet are unaware of interactions of herbal or other therapies and are ill equipped to assess the objective evidence for different types of complementary therapy. Such therapies, not provided by the NHS or by health insurance, can be costly and may be harmful, so the chapter on adjustment disorders is particularly useful in reviewing strategies for anxiety control and in looking at the ways that patients cope with the stress of adjusting to their situation.

Many patients are thought to be appropriately sad when they face their own dying, yet are actually clinically depressed and would benefit from pharmacological intervention. This book explores the difficulties in making a diagnosis of depression and also explores the problems and challenges posed by other psychiatric conditions in the patient receiving palliative care. Different interventions can assume that anyone with a little training can provide the necessary care; the importance of psychiatry and clinical psychology in the management of terminally ill patients and those facing a life-threatening illness has tended to be underestimated. The psychological management of a patient needs to be carefully arranged whether in the primary, secondary, or tertiary care sector. The availability of liaison psychiatry is variable around the UK; some units have well-defined links with other local services but in other areas there are unrealistic waiting lists or simply too few specialist trained staff to allow a service to be offered. The chapters on psychiatric disorders will help a professional know what to expect from a service and how to refer appropriately. When depression or hopelessness become severe, the will to live can give way to the wish to hasten death. When the tragedy of suicide occurs, the anger for the family and the sense of failure for them and the staff can be very difficult to cope with. The patient at risk of suicide must be detected and provided with the support to make their life tolerable. Suicide can be an angry act, which leaves the family much more deeply scarred than they would have been if death had occurred in a timely way.

The whole area of bereavement care is fraught with controversy. Some advocate less input from professionals, others advocate more. This book explores the reality of the tools available to measure outcomes of bereavement support and discusses the pros and cons of different models of support to the bereaved. The child facing bereavement has many practical and other concerns, including the legal frameworks required in arranging guardianship; all have to be addressed with sensitivity and accuracy. Children often do not have the opportunity to talk through their feelings with an adult who can really help them; their questions go unasked and therefore unanswered and many cultural myths prevent the child being included in the process of grieving with the rest of the family. It is crucial that all healthcare professionals understand children's responses to grief and loss and are able to support those adults who are the direct carers of the child.

It is not only cancer patients who need psychosocial support; it has been said that the cancer patient is lucky, as there are so many services available for those with cancer compared with other patient groups. Yet dying from a neurological disorder must seem infinitely frustrating and hard to come to terms with. Dying from cardiac failure carries with it the uncertainty of time and prognosis—such patients have particular needs.

This book should leave the reader feeling better equipped to deal with these complex issues and able to provide better-informed care.

Preface

I was introduced to palliative care as an elective student and almost immediately knew this was the area in which I wished to specialize.

During the past 12 years, I have learnt many things, the most important being that caring for patients with a terminal illness and their families requires the skills of many professionals working together as a team. However, it is often the psychosocial issues surrounding patients and families that cause individual members, and sometimes whole teams, the greatest difficulty. The issues of psychosocial assessment, treatment, care, and support of palliative care patients differ from the care of patients with early, treatable cancer—time is short and the emphasis different both from a patient and carer perspective.

This book is written in the hope that it will provide its readers with a new understanding of many of the issues of providing effective psychosocial care.

Many people have helped with the writing of this book. I wish to acknowledge the support of my former colleagues from the Leicestershire Hospice (LOROS). I was privileged to work at LOROS for six years and will be forever indebted to all the staff and volunteers who showed me what true teamworking could achieve and showed me what effective psychosocial care really means. Margaret Gold, art therapist, not only gave me new insights into art therapy but also allowed me and the readers to share in some of the work of the patients.

Catherine Barnes my editor from Oxford University Press has been an inspiring and enthusiastic friend over the last two years. I am deeply grateful to Baroness Finlay of Llandaff for writing the foreword—few people can be as busy and yet always find time to respond to requests for help. Michael Kearney has provided much supportive encouragement with this book and so many other things. Jennifer Barraclough gave me the initial encouragement to think about this book and has continued to give much ongoing support. I would like to thank Tony Armstrong Frost and Margaret Sanderson for sharing with me their experiences as carers and Isabel for allowing her thoughts to be incorporated into this book. Many other colleagues—Sam Ahmedzai, Yvonne Carter, Rob George, Geoff Hanks, Richard Hillier, Sheila Payne, Frances Sheldon, Fritz Stiefel, Trevor Friedman, Robert Twycross, and Andrew Wilcock have all given me unstinting support and encouragement. My colleagues at Liverpool Medical School have shown great interest and support, especially Chris Dowrick.

This book would never have been written without the inspiration of my patients. To share and accompany others on the last part of this earthly journey is one of the greatest privileges anyone can have. I have been humbled, inspired, and learnt so much from so many patients who would describe themselves as just ordinary people but who have shown extraordinary courage in the face of great adversity.

Mari Lloyd-Williams
Director of Community Studies
at the University of Liverpool Medical School

and

Consultant in Palliative Medicine
at Liverpool Marie Curie Centre and
Royal Liverpool Hospital

Contents

List of Plates

List of contributors

Ruth Benor, Psychotherapist, Devon, UK.

William Breitbart, Chief of Psychiatry Services, Department of Psychiatry, Memorial Sloan Kettering Hospital, New York, USA.

Mark Cobb, Chaplain and Clinical Director, Royal Hallamshire Hospital, Sheffield, UK.

Cathy Heaven, Communication Skills Tutor, CRC Psychological Medicine Group, Christie Hospital, Manchester, UK.

David Jeffrey, Macmillan Consultant in Palliative Medicine, Three Counties Cancer Centre, Cheltenham, UK.

Peter Maguire, Professor of Psychiatry, CRC Psychological Medicine Group, Christie Hospital, Manchester, UK.

Rod Macleod, Director of Palliative Care, Mary Potter Hospice, Wellington, New Zealand.

Steve Passik, Director Oncology Symptom Control Research, Indianapolis, USA.

Kenneth Kirsh, Research Scientist, University of Kentucky, USA.

Sheila Payne, Professor of Palliative Care Nursing, University of Sheffield, Sheffield, UK.

Hayley Pessin, Research Associate, Department of Psychiatry, Memorial Sloan Kettering Hospital, New York, USA.

Mordecai Potash, Clinical Psychiatry Fellow, Department of Psychiatry, Memorial Sloan Kettering Hospital, New York, USA.

Frances Sheldon, Macmillan Senior Lecturer in Social Work, University of Southampton, UK.

Leslie Walker, Director Institute of Rehabilitation, University of Hull, Hull, UK.

Donald Sharp, Senior Lecturer in Behavioural Oncology, Hull Cancer Centre, Hull, UK.

Mary Walker, Senior Clinical Nurse Specialist, Hull Oncology Support Centre, Hull, UK.

Mary Vachon, Associate Professor in Department of Psychiatry and Public Health, University of Toronto, Toronto, Canada.

Chapter 1

What do we mean by psychosocial care in palliative care?

David Jeffrey

Defining palliative care

Historically, hospice care developed as a response to perceived inadequacies in the care of dying patients and their families (Clark 2002). The pioneering work of hospices such as St Christopher's Hospice, which opened in 1967, demonstrated that the principles of hospice care could be applied in a variety of settings. Saunders introduced the concept of 'total pain', which highlighted not only the physical aspects of the patient's pain, but also the psychological, social, and spiritual dimensions of the patient's distress, which can all contribute to their suffering (Saunders 1993). The term 'palliative care' was coined in 1974 to reflect the extension of the discipline into mainstream medicine. In 1987, the Royal College of Physicians recognized palliative care as a specialty within medicine in the UK.

The World Health Organization's (WHO's) definition of palliative care was produced in 1990 (World Health Organization 1990):

> Palliative care is the active total care of patients whose disease is not responsive to curative treatment. Control of pain, of other symptoms and of psychological, social and spiritual problems is paramount. The goal of palliative care is achievement of the best quality of life for patients and their families. Many aspects of palliative care are also applicable earlier in the course of the illness, in conjunction with anticancer treatment.

Palliative care

(1) affirms life and regards dying as a normal process;

(2) neither hastens nor postpones death;

(3) provides relief from pain and other symptoms;

(4) integrates the psychological and spiritual aspects of patient care;

(5) offers a support system to help patients live as actively as possible until death;

(6) offers a support system to help the family cope during the patient's illness and in their own environment.

The definition now needs clarification. 'Total care', in the definition, refers to the holistic approach to the care of the patient. It does not mean that specialist palliative care services should take over the total care of the patient. Specialist palliative care services act as a resource to the primary professional carers. Furthermore, it may not be possible to 'control' psychological, social, or spiritual problems, as the definition seems to suggest. It is crucial however that these dimensions of care are assessed and addressed as far as possible.

The scope of palliative care extends beyond a patient with a diagnosis of cancer to include patients with other chronic life-threatening diseases. The statement 'neither hastens nor postpones death' reflects the philosophy of palliative care which rejects active euthanasia as a means of relieving suffering (National Council for Hospice and Specialist Palliative Care Services (NCHSPCS) 2002) Palliative treatments may lengthen survival, but it is not their primary goal, which is to improve quality of life.

Taking these reservations into account, the WHO definition of palliative care is applicable to palliative care delivered by any health or social care professional. Attempts have subsequently been made to clarify generic palliative care (or a palliative approach) and to distinguish it from specialist palliative care.

Generic palliative care services

A generic palliative care service comprises all the patient's and family's usual health-care professionals who provide palliative care as an integral part of their routine clinical practice. This practice is based on the following principles.

1. A focus on quality of life, which includes good symptom control. There is a need to assess what quality of life means for the individual patient. Patients are the experts on what gives quality to their own lives. The needs of patients change as the disease progresses so continual review is required.

2. A whole-person approach, taking into account the person's past life experience and current situation. Saunders's concept of total pain lies at the heart of palliative care.

3. Care which encompasses both the person with the life-threatening illness and those that matter to that person.

4. Respect for patient autonomy and choice. However, patients should not be forced to be autonomous when they do not wish to be (Sheldon 1997).

5. Emphasis on open and sensitive communication, which extends to patients, informal carers, and professional colleagues

The professional carers should be able to

(1) assess the palliative care needs of the patient and their family across the domains of physical, psychological, social, and spiritual need;

(2) meet those needs within the limits of their knowledge, skills, and competence;

(3) know when to seek advice from or refer to specialist palliative care services.

Professionals working in palliative care share common values and virtues: respect for patients to be self-determining within the limits of the rights of others, empathy and compassion, a sense of balance between hope and acceptance, and self-awareness. Palliative care is not highly technological but it is highly sophisticated and challenges practitioners on personal, clinical, and ethical levels.

Specialist palliative care services

Specialist palliative care services can be defined in terms of their core service components, their functions, and the composition of the multi-professional teams that deliver the service, which is underpinned by the same set of principles as generic palliative care services. The National Institute for Clinical Excellence has been commissioned by the Department of Health to provide guidance on supportive and palliative care. The National Council for Hospice and Specialist Palliative Care Services (2002) consultation paper anticipates that the following will be included as core service components of specialist palliative care:

- in-patient care
- community care
- day therapy
- hospital support
- bereavement services
- education.

A multi-professional specialist palliative care team delivers specialist palliative care. Members of this team will include

- specialist nursing staff
- a consultant in palliative medicine
- a social worker
- a clinical psychologist
- an occupational therapist
- a physiotherapist
- a chaplain or other religious leader.

The complexity of the issues raised by patients and their families demands a team approach, because no individual could meet all the needs. The specialist palliative care services include National Health Service (NHS) and voluntary sector providers who make up the supportive and palliative care network serving a local health community.

Psychosocial care

The National Council for Hospice and Specialist Palliative Care Services (1997) has defined psychosocial care as

> concerned with the psychological and emotional well being of the patient and their family/carers, including issues of self-esteem, insight into an adaptation to the illness and its consequences, communication, social functioning and relationships.

Psychosocial care addresses the psychological experiences of loss and facing death for the patient and their impact on those close to them. It involves the spiritual beliefs, culture, and values of those concerned and the social factors that influence the experience. Psychosocial care includes the practical aspects of care such as financial, housing, and aids to daily living, and overlaps with spiritual care. Spiritual care is less easy to define but includes emotional benefits of informal support from relatives, friends, religious groups, and more formal pastoral care.

Psychosocial care also involves professional carers who are inevitably affected by their experiences and who thus require support.

Thus psychosocial care encompasses

(1) psychological approaches, which are concerned with enabling patients and those close to them to express thoughts, feelings, and concerns relating to illness;

(2) psychological interventions to improve the psychological and emotional well-being of the patient and their family and carers.

In the past there has been greater emphasis on psychological needs than social needs—the National Council for Hospice and Specialist Palliative Care Services (2000) have emphasized the importance of social care to patients:

> The social fabric of their lives is central to how they make sense of their illness experiences, the meanings they draw upon to understand these and the range of resources they can call upon to help them manage them.

In practice, the social aspects of palliative care are often limited to a focus upon the patient's family, ignoring community influences.

The NCHSPCS discussion paper suggests that we might replace the term 'psychosocial care' with 'psychological care' and 'social care' to emphasize the importance of social care and community issues of culture and ethnicity (National Council for Hospice and Specialist Palliative Care 1995).

Patients may feel a sense of loss of control, fear, or anger when confronted by a terminal illness (Plate 1, pp. 98–99). Their relatives too may be experiencing these emotions and the sad consequence is that this often causes a distancing between them. Helping patients and families to express emotions can reduce fear and anxiety and help to bridge family relationships. Spiritual issues extend beyond the religious to include existential issues around the meaning of an individual's life; again, giving people the opportunity to address these concerns helps to alleviate suffering. Practical help can empower patients to be involved in decision making and to exercise choice. If patients and families feel involved in decision making they have a greater sense of control.

Good palliative care and therefore good psychosocial care depends upon effective teamwork. Individual members of the team have overlapping roles and overlapping skills. Each profession within the team brings its own perspective. Psychosocial care focuses on both the patient's 'journey' and the 'journeys' of their family and friends as members of a community.

The boundaries of psychosocial care are unclear. For example, physical care such as washing and bathing a patient may have effects on the patient's mood, self-esteem, and feelings of dependency. Similarly, attending to a practical concern such as making a will may lead to a reduction in anxiety. There is a huge overlap in psychological and spiritual care when listening to existential concerns such as 'Why me?'. The situation is made more complex because the patient may choose to confide their concerns to any member of the team; so, for example, it may be the district nurse who has to deal with questions about the meaning of the illness or anxieties about dying.

Supportive care

The development of the NHS Cancer Plan (Department of Health 2000) led to the terms 'palliative care' and 'supportive care', terms used to reflect the holistic and multi-professional dimensions of this area of care. The purpose of the Cancer Plan is to ensure that people with cancer get the right professional support and care as well as the best treatment. The Cancer Plan envisaged the development of palliative and supportive care networks that are to sit alongside cancer networks. The debate has now moved towards differentiating between supportive and palliative care.

Defining supportive care

Supportive care refers to care that is designed to help the patient and their family cope with cancer and its treatment at all stages of the cancer journey. It helps the patient to maximize the benefits of treatment and to live as well as possible with the effects of the disease.

The key principles underpinning good supportive care comprise

- a focus on quality of life
- a whole-person approach
- care to include the patient and those who matter to the patient
- respect for patient autonomy and choice
- an emphasis on open and sensitive communication.

The principal needs addressed by supportive care include information, integrated-support-service, humanity, empowerment, physical, continuity-of-care, psychological, social, and spiritual needs.

Clearly there are areas of overlap between supportive and palliative care and the debate on the definitions will continue. It is important that generic services can assess needs and know when to refer and that a range of specialist palliative care services exist to complement the generic service.

Palliative care in different settings

Palliative care is applicable in most settings. However in the UK almost a quarter of occupied hospital bed days are taken up by patients who are in the last year of life. In the UK, 60% of all deaths take place in hospital, despite a strong patient preference for dying at home (Townsend et al. 1990). Seymour (2001) has commented on the social isolation of dying patients in hospital and of the failure of medical technology to coexist appropriately with dignified dying. Mola (1997) found that hospital is often perceived to be a place of insecurity, discomfort, intrusion, and demands for compliance. This can be contrasted with the home setting where generally there is a sense of social and physical security and where sick people may have a greater sense of control. The patient's privacy can be threatened when the many different professional carers visit the home in an uncoordinated way. We need to question the extent to which patient preferences are taken into account in treatment decisions to avoid medicalizing the home, because it seems that as far as palliative care services are concerned the wishes of the users are at variance with the policies of the providers (Clark *et al.* 1997). However, by listening to patients and those close to them, the nature of appropriate care becomes clear. Mola has identified circumstances that influence care of the dying:

- a favourable family environment
- acceptance of death
- supportive family
- availability of voluntary carers
- patient's preferences a priority.

Douglas (1992) challenged the hospice movement when he asked 'Why should only the minority who die of malignancies—and precious few even of them, be singled out for deluxe dying?'

When should palliative care start?

For cancer patients, palliative care may start at diagnosis, although it is more usual to start when cure is no longer possible (Regnard and Kindlen 2001). There is a trend towards moving palliative care to earlier in the patient's journey thus shifting the focus away from terminal care. This trend is linked to the desire to extend the benefits of palliative care to those with diseases other than cancer, thus broadening the boundaries of palliative care.

Currently there is confusion within this specialty that relates to a stage of disease rather than pathology. Furthermore there is no clear guidance as to the relationship between palliative and supportive care. Clark (2002) states that the challenge facing palliative care is how to reconcile the high expectations of technical expertise with calls for a humanistic and ethical orientation to the care. There is a concern to understand what is best practice and what the experience is like for the patient, carer, and professional. Psychosocial aspects of palliative care have to be the concern of all the team because all the elements comprising total pain require attention if suffering is to be relieved and quality of life improved.

Psychosocial assessment

Patients and families face a range of issues that are not only related to illness and approaching death. The healthcare professionals need to assess individual strengths, coping styles, experience, and stress and attend to previous losses.

The initial assessment of a patient is carried out by a member of the specialist palliative care team and will include a detailed medical and nursing assessment of the patient's, family's, and carers' needs. The time invested in this initial assessment is not wasted but builds a firm foundation for the patient–professional partnership. The initial assessment may indicate the need for more formal psychological or social assessment (Monroe 1998). This will include the following domains

(1) the need to maintain autonomy, which includes respect for dignity and the opportunity to exercise choice;

(2) the need for psychological, social, and spiritual support.

We need to assess the ways in which the illness has changed the life of the individual, their coping strategies, and their sources of support. Discussion of their hopes and expectations will identify any unfinished business. The impact of the disease on their relationships and concepts of body image may identify psychosexual issues which need addressing.

We need to explore both the losses incurred in the present illness and to understand the patient's previous bereavements. The assessment should include a discussion of the meaning of the illness to the patient and to the family. This will include a review of the patient's hopes and fears for the future and their expectations.

1. **Family issues.** Much of this information can be summarized on a genogram or family tree. We need to gain an insight into how the family functions, the conflicts, and vulnerable individuals. We need to understand the family roles and and how these have changed as a result of the illness.

2. **The need for practical help.** Physical resources such as money and housing. Physical needs, independence, mobility, toileting, and sleeping. Adaptations to the home and provision of support may avoid the need for in-patient care.

3. **Social issues.** The family's perspective needs to be placed in the context of their community. The team needs to understand its ethnic, cultural, and religious background and the potential impact of these influences on the individual and their family and carers. These assessments should be based on an understanding of loss and change, family dynamics, communication, counselling, and knowledge of social policy and resources.

Screening and assessment scales

In addition to the general assessment of psychosocial needs there are also a number of assessment scales, which are tools to measure specific aspects of psychological symptoms or quality of life. For example, the hospital anxiety and depression scale (HAD) (Zigmond and Snaith 1983) and the overall quality of life scales (Morgan 2000). The patient's involvement is central as they are the experts on what factors give quality to their lives. There are methodological problems in assessing and measuring quality of life in patients with advanced cancer. Whilst the range of current measures provides researchers and clinicians with a choice, the existence of so many different assessment scales reflects the underlying methodological uncertainty.

On the basis of the assessment the team may suggest interventions to the patient and family but needs to be sensitive to the fact that patients are experts too and may have views that differ from the professional team. We need to have the humility to listen and to respect the patient's need for privacy.

Psychosocial interventions

Healthcare staff should all provide psychosocial care in the broad sense. Psychosocial support means care which enhances well-being, confidence, and social functioning. Specialist psychosocial care is the provision within specialist palliative care of staff who are appropriately trained and qualified in psychosocial interventions and the holistic assessment of needs of patients and their families. These staff provide psychosocial and practical care and advice or supervision of psychosocial care by other staff. Psychologists, social workers, and chaplains, who share key skills, provide such specialist care.

Psychological interventions

These may include a range of interventions and support to relieve symptoms such as anxiety or anger, or to recognize and treat specific psychiatric disorders such as depression.

These interventions may be offered to the patient, family, or bereaved individuals, to improve the psychological and emotional well-being of the patient and their family and carers.

Examples of psychological interventions include (Chochinov and Breitbart 2000)

◆ psychosocial support and psychotherapy;
◆ behavioural–cognitive therapies;
◆ educational therapies.

Psychological therapies are used increasingly in palliative care. Techniques such as cognitive and behavioural therapies have been adapted from the arena of mental health for use in cancer patients who are suffering from anxiety, low mood, or stress (Moorey and Greer 1989). These therapies explore patients' existing coping strategies and facilitate the development of new and effective strategies so that patients regain a sense of control. Guided imagery is another technique to aid relaxation (Kearney 1992). Others have used patient narratives to encourage reminiscence and to encourage a holistic approach by gaining insights into the patient's world.

Social interventions

The specialist social worker in the team may be involved in a range of interventions involving patients, families, carers, and the local community. These include

(1) providing information to patients and families about the resources available and arranging practical help, which includes acting as an advocate for the patient to enable access to financial benefits or legal advice;

(2) liaison with local and national statutory and voluntary agencies;

(3) organizing packages of care at home or negotiating placement and securing funding for residential nursing home care;

(4) identifying people at special risk in bereavement and ensuring appropriate support is available.

Social care involves the identification and mobilization of resources that will help the patient, family, and carers cope with the situation whether these are resources within the family or resources produced by NHS statutory or voluntary agencies.

One feature of multi-professional teamwork is the blurring of roles and nowhere is this more prevalent than in the provision of psychosocial care. For example, bereavement support of the family may be undertaken by a social worker, a clinical psychologist, or a clinical nurse specialist. The team needs to be aware that there is a risk of overwhelming the patient or their family with support so care must be coordinated. The overlapping boundaries of psychosocial care may cause difficulties for professionals within the team and there is a risk that some members may feel undervalued.

Staff support

To gain insight into the unique world of the individual patient requires an effort of empathy. The needs and fears of patients facing death make us confront our own vulnerability and may make professionals feel inadequate. A psychological challenge for professionals is to learn to live with these negative feelings and to continue to support the patient, family, and carers.

Management in ensuring adequate resources, such as accommodation, staffing levels, administrative support, and annual and study leave can support professional teams. Stress leads to absenteeism and further stress for remaining team members culminating in staff 'burning out'. We need to value and nurture skilled professionals. Practical means of support include skilled team leadership, debriefing sessions, and individual supervision and appraisal. Support should not be restricted to paid staff but should include volunteers.

Psychiatry and palliative care

It is important that any psychosocial assessment is able to distinguish between an appropriate response to a life-threatening illness and the symptoms of a psychiatric disorder. Treating psychiatric morbidity in patients with advanced cancer improves their quality of life (Macmillan Practice Development Unit 1996). The most common psychiatric disorders are depression and abnormal grieving and anxiety states. Furthermore specialist psychiatric help may also be required for patients with existing psychiatric disorders who develop a terminal illness such as cancer.

Depression is the most common psychiatric problem in the palliative setting (Lloyd-Williams and Friedman 2001). Its definition as a diagnostic treatable clinical syndrome is not clear cut. It occurs as a continuum of severity of depressive symptoms and somewhere along this continuum clinicians make decisions as to when treatment is appropriate. Depression in patients with advanced cancer is underdiagnosed and may not be appropriately treated, thus impairing the patient's quality of life. More effective methods of diagnosing depression are needed in palliative care.

Both psychological and pharmacological treatments are effective in patients with severe depression. Professionals need to have a high index of suspicion for depression, particularly for younger patients with advanced disease.

Why is psychosocial care so important?

It is important for the psychosocial needs of the patient and carers to be assessed so that appropriate levels of support and treatment can be offered. A psychosocial approach is a patient-and-family-centred approach and is vitally important as it represents a mechanism for retaining the holistic approach of modern palliative care. Psychosocial care can restore many of the original values and visions of palliative care to a specialty threatened by increasing medical technology.

Clark (2002) identifies four key strands in modern palliative care:

(1) a shift in the literature on care of the dying from anecdote to systematic observation and research;

(2) a new openness about the terminal condition of patients with concepts of dignity and meaning;

(3) an active rather than passive approach to care of the dying;

(4) a growing recognition of the interdependency of mental and physical distress, notions of suffering, and the concept of total pain.

However just when it seems that palliative care has persuaded doctors to be gentler in their acceptance of death, the influence of advancing medical technology has led to the adoption of futile treatments and an assumption in society that every cause of death can be resisted, postponed, or avoided. The integration of specialist palliative care into mainstream medicine risks medicalization of the specialty. The process of medicalization implies that the biomedical model replaces the holistic caring approach that defined the early development of the specialty. In a biomedical model, symptoms are equated with suffering, the focus of care is the malfunctioning of organs, and there is a perceived need for pharmacological control of symptoms. Furthermore, even the concept of total pain, intended to emphasize a holistic approach, risks being split into component parts. Thus in a specialist palliative care team there is a risk that if the biomedical model is applied, the consultant would address symptoms with medication, which would be regarded as the most important part of care, whilst the social worker would deal with patient finances and allowances, the nurse with physical care, and the psychologist or psychiatrist with the patient's worries. This biomedical approach risks ignoring concepts such as suffering and denying our common humanity (Dunlop and Hockley 1997).

The assessment of psychosocial needs seeks to understand the patient's interpretation of their illness and assist them in constructing a new understanding. Suffering is the key issue to be addressed. Its complex nature demands a team approach to support and care (Vachon 1998).

We need to regain the sense of a 'good death' and restore our expectations of how long we live to patterns of community life and a sense of an appropriate time for our life to end rather than place unrealistic demands upon medical technology (Fraser 2002). If we have no idea of what a good death might be how can we articulate our fears and emotional distress? Patients and their families want to be treated with humanity; they need information and want to be involved in decisions relating to their health as much as in any other domain of their life.

References

Chochinov HM, Breitbart W (ed.) (2000). *Handbook of psychiatry in palliative medicine.* Oxford: Oxford University Press, p. 25.

Clark D (2000). Between hope and acceptance: the medicalisation of dying. *BMJ* 324:905–7.

Clark D, Hockley J, Ahmedzai S (1997). *New themes in palliative care.* Buckingham: Open University Press.

Corner J, Dunlop R (1997). New approaches to care. In: Clark D, Hockley J, Ahmedzai S (ed.). *New themes in palliative care.* Buckingham: Open University Press, p. 289.

Department of Health (2000). *The NHS cancer plan.* London: Her Majesty's Stationery Office.

Douglas C (1992). For all the saints. *BMJ* 304:579.

Fraser G (2002). Estranged from death. *The Guardian* 10 May 2002.

Kearney M (1992). Image work in a case of intractable pain. *Palliative Med* 2:152–7.

Lloyd-Williams M, Friedman T (2001). Depression in palliative care patients—a prospective study. *Eur J Cancer Care* 10:270–4.

Macmillan Practice Development Unit (1996). *Anxiety and depression in cancer and palliative care: a nursing perspective.* London: Cancer Relief Macmillan Fund.

Mola GD (1997). Palliative home care. In: Clark D, Hockley J, Ahmedzai S (ed.). *New themes in palliative care.* Buckingham: Open University Press, pp. 129–42.

Monroe B (1998). Social work in palliative care. In: Doyle D, Hanks G , MacDonald N (ed.). 2nd edn. *Oxford textbook of palliative medicine.* Oxford: Oxford University Press, p. 867.

Moorey S, Greer S (1989). *Psychological therapy with cancer patients: a new approach.* Oxford: Heinemann Medical.

Morgan G (2000). Assessment of quality of life in palliative care. *Int J Palliative Care Nursing* 6:406–9.

National Council for Hospice and Specialist Palliative Care (1995). Opening doors: improving access to hospice and specialist palliative care services by members of the black and ethic minority communities. London; January 1995. Occasional Paper No. 7.

National Council for Hospice and Specialist Palliative Care Services (1997). Feeling better: psychosocial care in specialist palliative care. London; April 1997. Occasional Paper No. 13.

National Council for Hospice and Specialist Palliative Care Services (2000). What do we mean by 'psychosocial'? London; March 2000. Briefing No. 4.

National Council for Hospice and Specialist Palliative Care Services (2002). Definitions of supportive and palliative care. London; January 2002. A consultation paper.

Regnard C, Kindlen M (2001). *What is palliative care? Current learning in palliative care (CLIP).* Newcastle upon Tyne: St Oswald's Hospice.

Saunders C, Sykes (ed.) (1993). *The management of terminal malignant disease*. London: Edwards Arnold.

Seymour JE (2001). *Critical moments—death and dying in intensive care*. Buckingham: Open University Press.

Sheldon F (1997). *Psychosocial palliative care*. Cheltenham: Stanley Thornes Ltd, p. 5–14.

Townsend J, Frank AO, Fermont D, Karran O, Walgrave A Piper M (1990). Terminal cancer and patients preference for place of death: a prospective study. *BMJ* **301**:415–17.

Vachon M (1998) The emotional problems of the patient. In: Doyle D, Hanks G , MacDonald N (ed.). 2nd edn. *Oxford textbook of palliative medicine*. Oxford: Oxford University Press, p. 919.

World Health Organization (1990). Cancer pain relief and palliative care. Geneva. Report of a WHO expert committee.

Zigmond AS, Snaith RP (1983). The hospital anxiety and depression scale. *Acta Psychiat Scand* **67**:361–70.

Chapter 2

Communication issues

Cathy Heaven and Peter Maguire

Introduction

This chapter reviews the problems that health professionals involved in cancer and palliative care report in communicating with patients, families, and colleagues. A three-step
guide to improving practice is presented, which is both evidence based and practical:

(1) understanding how communication goes wrong and considering why this happens;

(2) identifying the key skills necessary for effective interviewing and the criteria to use
when assessing the likely effectiveness of training courses;

(3) addressing how skills can be applied within clinical practice and maintained over
time.

The need to improve communication skills within palliative care

There is a strong link between the number and severity of patients' concerns and
the later development of anxiety and depression. Weisman and Worden (1997) first
reported a link between concerns and emotional distress; more recently the connection between concerns and psychiatric morbidity was demonstrated in newly diagnosed (Parle *et al.* 1996) and palliative care patients (Heaven and Maguire 1998) and
in relatives or carers of cancer patients (Pitceathly *et al.* 2000). A relationship has also
been established between the types of concerns commonly found in palliative care,
like pain (Derogatis *et al.* 1983), fatigue, (Worden and Weisman 1977), and breathlessness (Bredin *et al.* 1999) and psychiatric morbidity.

Given that one in three cancer patients suffers from an episode of anxiety or depression regardless of stage (Razavi *et al.* 1990; Ibbotson *et al.* 1994; Fulton 1998) and
between 30 and 33 per cent of relatives also suffer an episode of such morbidity
(Pitceathly *et al.* 2000; Kissane *et al.* 1994), it is vital that healthcare professionals are
able to identify concerns and recognize the associated distress. However, in practice,
many concerns are not elicited (Heaven and Maguire 1997). This failure to elicit problems is not restricted to the psychological domain but also applies to physical concerns,

for example, pain (Glajchen *et al.* 1995). In a recent study it was established that only 20 per cent of patients concerns within palliative care were elicited and identified (Heaven and Maguire 1997). Consequently many patients are not given the appropriate help or support to resolve or come to terms with their difficulties.

It has been found that patients cope better with their predicament if they perceive they are given adequate information (Butow *et al.* 1996). Yet only a small proportion receive the information they require (Hinds *et al.* 1995); patients given too much or too little information are at an increased risk of anxiety and depression (Fallowfield *et al.* 1990). The challenge for the health professional is to establish what information patients need; however, many do not have the strategies to do this (Suominen *et al.* 1994; Ford *et al.* 1996) and tend to use routine ways of giving the information, which take no account of individual needs or preferences (Maguire 1998).

Patient involvement in decision making can lead to dissatisfaction and non-compliance (Dowsett *et al.* 2000) and affect patient outcomes adversely (Coulter 1999). There is some debate as to whether all seriously ill cancer patients want involvement in decision making (Cox 2002). Rothenbacher *et al.* (1997) established that the majority of patients with advanced cancer want a collaborative or active role in decisions but a substantial minority (28%) desire a passive role. Thus, healthcare professionals need to identify those who wish to take part in decisions and respect those who wish the clinician to take decisions for them. Clinicians do not know how to assess patients' wish for involvement (Rothenbacher *et al.* 1997) and fear patients will blame themselves or lose confidence in the doctor if treatment does not work (Richards *et al.* 1995). Doctors can take refuge in a paternalistic approach, in which less disclosure and less patient participation are favoured (Fallowfield *et al.* 1990; de Valch *et al.* 2001) but this increases both anxiety and depression (Morris and Royle 1987; Ashcroft *et al.* 1985).

These communication difficulties create problems for patients and relatives and also affect healthcare professionals. Lack of confidence in their ability to communicate with patients and relatives contributes to high levels of burn-out in cancer professionals (Delvaux *et al.* 1988; Ramirez *et al.* 1996). A study of 882 consultants (Ramirez *et al.* 1996) established a link between those who felt insufficiently trained in communication skills and higher levels of emotional exhaustion and depersonalization and lower levels of personal accomplishment. The consultants reported that their training had not equipped them with the relevant communication skills. Within palliative care and oncology nursing, communication problems have been identified as contributory factors to stress, burn-out, illness, and staff turnover (Baider and Porath 1981; Grey-Toft and Anderson 1981).

Many health professionals report frustration in communicating with colleagues (Maguire and Faulkner 1988; Fallowfield *et al.* 1990) but little research has been conducted in this area. A study of 48 nurses showed that much of the written interprofessional reporting was task orientated, focused on medical treatments, and failed to cover psychological and social aspects of care (Dowding 2001). The study also showed that during shift reports nurses recorded less than half the information given or discussed, and recalled less than 27 per cent. There was a clear bias in recall towards medical information, treatment, and history. Professionals appear to only report and record a small amount of the information they have elicited from the patient (Heaven and Maguire 1997).

Summary

Within palliative care there are a number of key communication tasks. The importance of accurately assessing patients' concerns and worries, tailoring information to patients' needs, and involving patients in decision making have all been highlighted, as well as communicating these aspects to colleagues. Deficits in these key areas lead to problems for patients and relatives, and also healthcare professionals, as they recognize and worry about their inability to deliver best-quality care.

Improving communication

The key to improving communication is to understand how and why it breaks down. Only then can health professionals begin to develop more effective communication behaviours.

Step 1: understanding how and why communication breaks down

How communication breaks down

Healthcare professionals often 'distance' from what the patient is saying. While this is often a conscious process (Booth *et al.* 1996) it may also happen unconsciously (Maguire 1985). From analysis of many consultations (Maguire *et al.* 1996) behaviours that have the function of distancing have been identified.

Selective attention

This happens when the interviewer controls the content of the conversation by picking up only certain areas, commonly those which are factual or which contain no feeling. In doing this the interviewer limits the agenda to those topics they feel comfortable discussing or helping with. For example,

> Patient: 'I was in pain, weak, and tired and was absolutely terrified that the treatment wasn't working.'
>
> Interviewer: 'Tell me about your pain. How bad was it?'

It is of note that this type of behaviour has been reported in both nurses (Crow *et al.* 1995) and doctors (Bornstein and Emler 2001).

Switching

Switching is the term used when the interviewer changes the focus of what is being said, so controlling the content, emotional depth, or focus of the conversation. Switching can happen in several ways.

1. **Switching the time focus.** This is when the interviewer moves the 'time-frame' of the interview, so preventing the patient from, for example, talking about initial fears, by encouraging them to focus on current thoughts. In doing this, the interviewer

inhibits patients from expressing their emotions about past events, by focusing them on different events.

Patient: 'It was awful, I felt so ill, and so fed up, it seemed to go on for ever.'

Interviewer: 'And how do you feel now?'

2. **Switching the topic.** This is when the interviewer, often unconsciously, changes the topic or content of the conversation completely.

Patient: 'I have been having some pain, it worries me somewhat.'

Interviewer: 'How has your breathing been?'

3. **Switching the person focus.** This happens when the interviewer changes the focus of the interview from the interviewee, or person being spoken to, to a third party, either present at the interview or not, so inhibiting the interviewee from talking about how they feel.

Patient: 'I felt devastated by the news. It thought I was going to die.'

Interviewer: 'And how did your wife feel about it?'

Offering advice or reassurance

One of the most common responses to expression of emotion is for health professionals to give reassurance or offer advice. However, Maguire *et al.* (1996) in their investigation of facilitative and inhibitory interviewing behaviours found that giving advice prematurely significantly decreased patient disclosure. The difficulty for most healthcare professionals is that they choose to enter their profession to help the individuals that they care for by solving their problems. Seeing a person in distress, or even worse, when distressing a person by delivering bad news, evokes in the majority of professionals the need to alleviate the distress and make the situation better.

Patient: 'I feel so shocked by the news.'

Interviewer: 'You will get over that feeling, it doesn't last for too long.'

Patient: I'm really worried about having pain, my father had pain you see.'

Interviewer: 'Please try not to worry about that. Not all people with cancer suffer pain and we have made wonderful advances since your father's day. We have many, many types of pain killers available to use'.

In each of these examples moving immediately into 'distress alleviation mode' has the function of inhibiting the patient from saying more about their distress or from clarifying the particular worry. This means that the health professional's advice or reassurance may not actually address the patient's real concern.

Using jargon

Using medical jargon in communication can create an obstacle between the patient or relative and the healthcare professional. It is interesting to note that the use of medical terminology is not confined solely to health professionals. As information is now widely available from the Internet there is increasing evidence that patients and relatives are using medical terms that may or may not be fully understood. Health professionals need to be alert not only to their own use of language but also to medical terms used by the patient, which may seem appropriate, but which may be a source of misunderstanding as the word may simply be being repeated without having been understood.

Passing the buck

Here the interviewer, in direct response to the patient's cue or concerns, advises the patient to talk to a third party. Whilst this may be appropriate at the end of an interview, using it immediately a patient mentions a problem indicates that the interviewer does not want to hear the patients concerns.

> Patient: 'I was so upset, I just didn't know what he meant.'

> Interviewer: 'Clearly you need to talk to the surgeon about that, to get things clear.'

Why communication breaks down

Effective communication is a complex process, dependent on a number of factors relating to both the professional and to the recipient of the communication. If communication is to be improved, these factors, summarized in Fig. 2.1 and illustrated in Fig. 2.2, must be acknowledged and understood (Bandura 1977). The health professional's personal attitudes and beliefs can have an impact on communication, as well as fears and the amount of support available within the working environment. The recipients are also affected by their own attitudes, beliefs, values, and fears.

One of the most illuminating studies in this area related nurses' explanations of their interviewing behaviours to actual instances of distancing (Booth *et al.* 1996) at the same time as exploring patients' reasons for non-disclosure (Heaven and Maguire 1997). The study was conducted in a hospice setting and investigated the interviewing behaviour of 41 nurses as they went through a 10-week communication skills training programme. The study involved all nursing staff, qualified and unqualified, at two hospices. The nurses conducted interviews with 87 patients and completed questionnaires

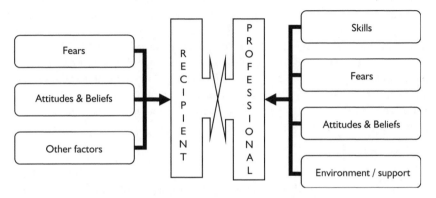

Fig. 2.1 Factors affecting health care professionals' communication.

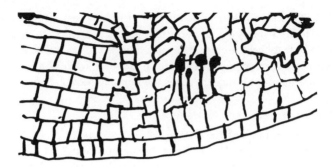

Fig. 2.2 Communication—The wall of silence.

to assess perceived support, and semi-structured interviews in which they were asked to talk about specific instances of distancing behaviour evident from recording their assessment interviews (Booth *et al.* 1996). The patients were interviewed using the concerns checklist and were questioned about disclosure (Heaven and Maguire 1997). In the majority of cases the nurses were conscious of their distancing behaviours and gave clear explanations as to why they had changed the focus or switched topic at the identified points. Patients were conscious of withholding information from the nurses and could also give cogent reasons (Heaven and Maguire 1997).

Professionals' lack of skills

One of the reasons why communication breaks down that was given by the nurses in the study of Booth *et al.* was their perception that they lacked skills. Studies of communication in medicine and nursing have shown repeatedly that doctors and nurses lack the skills necessary to elicit and explore patients' concerns and to identify and respond to patients' information needs and decision-making preferences (Maguire *et al.* 1996; Heaven and Maguire 1996; Razavi *et al.* 2000; Wilkinson *et al.* 1998; Fallowfield 2002).

Healthcare professionals experience other difficulties when interviewing, for example, integrating factual, physical, emotional, social, and spiritual modes of enquiry (Maguire *et al.* 1996), assessing less familiar aspects (such as body image or anxious preoccupation), and knowing how to close an interview which has been emotional (Parle *et al.* 1997). Coping with key tasks, for example, giving bad news about a poor prognosis, negotiating with a relative who wishes to withhold the truth from a patient, or supporting a dying patient (Fallowfield *et al.* 1998; Razavi *et al.* 2000; Maguire and Faulkner 1988) are also areas that clinicians find difficult. Other challenging communication tasks highlighted in the literature include handling difficult questions (Hitch and Murgatroyd 1983; Maguire and Faulkner 1988), dealing with anger (Duldt 1982; Smith and Hart 1994), and handling denial, collusion, and withdrawn and silent patients (Delveaux *et al.* 1988).

Professionals' fears

The second category of factors that affects communication is fear. The literature points to a large number of fears that affect health professionals' use of communication skills, many of which relate to palliative care (Heaven and Maguire 1997). These include fear of upsetting the patient and fear of unleashing strong emotions such as anger or uncontrollable distress. Many health professionals are aware of the depth and strength of patients' and relatives' emotions and so fear encouraging the expression of them; for example, asking how a patient feels when they have just been told they are dying could easily provoke extreme distress or even anger. If the professional giving the bad news is fearful of handling such emotions then the likelihood of giving the patient the chance to ventilate their feelings is remote.

Another fear is that of opening up a 'can of worms' and in doing so giving patients false expectations about professionals' ability to alleviate concerns. Health professionals may fear getting out of their depth or being unable to cope with the list of worries and may respond in a way that would make the situation worse for the patient or even damage the patient (Bond 1983; Maguire 1985; Booth *et al.* 1996).

Fear of taking up too much time is reported as a deterrent to exploring feelings by many nurses and doctors, who envisage that once patients are encouraged to talk about emotions they will be difficult to stop or they may somehow lose control (Maguire 1985; Fielding and Llewelyn 1987; Sellick 1991). Even in palliative care, where time is often less of an issue, the fear of getting stuck with a patient or of not being able to complete our allocated workload can be a powerful deterrent to exploring the concerns expressed (Booth *et al.* 1996).

In a study of in-depth interviews with general practitioners (GPs), Rosser and Maguire (1982) noted that the fear of having to face one's own sense of failure in not being able to help also influenced health professionals' willingness to talk openly with their patients (Rosser and Maguire 1982). This is echoed by Baider and Porath (1981) in discussing nurses' difficulties in facing patients who are having difficult death experiences. One's own death anxieties have been identified as a factor mediating communication with patients by a number of authors (Field and Kitson 1986; Wilkinson 1991; Tait 1994) and have therefore been part of a number of training schemes aimed at altering communication behaviours (Brown 1981; Rickert 1982; Razavi *et al.*1993).

It is easy to see how such strong fears about what might happen inhibit and change the course of an interview. If these issues are not explored and addressed they will inevitably result in professionals exhibiting 'blocking' behaviours to protect both the patient and themselves from what they perceive might be negative consequences (Razavi *et al.* 2000; Parle *et al.* 1997; Heaven and Maguire 1997).

Professionals' attitudes and beliefs

A broad number of attitudes have been associated with distancing. Beliefs about emotional problems being an inevitable consequence of a palliative situation encourages professionals to either ignore concerns or to normalize them, that is, to accept that everyone feels like that (Johnston 1982; Peterson 1988; Booth *et al.* 1996). This, coupled with the belief that nothing can be done about certain types of concerns (for example, anxiety whilst waiting for results), can mean some worries get overlooked or minimized (Hardman *et al.* 1989; Maguire 1985). There is evidence that nurses and doctors believe there is no point in talking about things which cannot be changed and that opening up irresolvable issues will upset the patient unnecessarily (Booth *et al.* 1996). In a palliative situation this might be shown by reluctance to discuss issues like 'what might happen when the cancer becomes worse'. The professional does this to protect the patient, who, realizing the health professional is reluctant to talk about them, remains isolated with their concerns.

The belief that people from different cultures experience different problems or interpret things differently can be a powerful deterrent to open communication. This may explain why cultural differences were put at the top of the list of patient characteristics that oncologists found most difficult to handle (Fallowfield *et al.* 1998). An awareness of cultural differences will enhance professional communication but evidence suggests that patients in different cultures experience similar worries and problems (Cheturvedi *et al.* 1996) and the same range of emotional difficulties (Kai-Hoi Sue *et al.* 2000) and that constructs like quality of life are stable across several cultural boundaries (Lo *et al.* 2001).

Beliefs that if patients have concerns they will volunteer them spontaneously can also hinder communication (Maguire 1985; Hardman *et al.* 1989), as can the notion that heathcare professionals should not intrude on patients' private feelings by asking directly about their fears and concerns (Booth *et al.* 1996).

Professionals' environment and support

The final factor known to affect health professionals' use of their communication is the environment in which they work. A direct link has been made between support and communication behaviour. Wilkinson (1991) studied the factors affecting the assessment skills of 56 ward nurses. She demonstrated that the main factor related to nurses' blocking behaviours was perceived support from the ward sister. Confirmation of the influence of the ward sister or senior members of staff comes from Peterson (1988), who found nurses highly influenced by the views of their colleagues, Moorhead and Winefield (1991), who identified the culture of senior staff as being highly influential in the communication skills that medical students used, and Booth *et al.* (1996), who identified the lack of availability of help when needed and supervisors not being perceived as concerned with the nurses' welfare as two major factors related to hospice nurses' blocking behaviours. Heaven (2001) showed that nurses who were unsupported after training were significantly less likely to use facilitative communication skills with their patients and more likely to respond to patient cues in a negative way.

Many authors have discussed the role of stress and support in determining communication behaviour (Hanson 1994; Larson 1993; Delvaux *et al.* 1988, Ramirez *et al.* 1996). McElroy (1982) in reviewing the literature in cancer nursing notes that

> Today the professional nurse realises the importance of giving emotional support and compassionate care to each patient and family. As a result of this involvement, the nurse is more vulnerable, and this adds to the stress already present in her job. The nurse who does not receive emotional support is not able to give emotional support.

Other influences created by the ward environment include a feeling of there being lack of time (Bond 1983; Macleod Clark 1983); however for evidence, the relationship of workload to communication behaviour shows that workload impacts on nurses' feelings of stress and that reducing workload is not associated with increased communication with the patients (Huckaby and Neal 1979).

Patient behaviours

The role of patients in breakdown of communication has already been acknowledged. As part of the training study already mentioned, hospice patients were interviewed to identify their concerns, after their nursing carers had assessed them (Heaven and Maguire 1997). Comparison of the patients' concerns list and a list generated from ratings of the audiotaped interviews revealed that the patients withheld up to 60% of the concerns they were experiencing. Patients experiencing most distress, as assessed by the hospital anxiety and depression scale, withheld most concerns. Content analysis demonstrated that patients were only revealing certain types of concerns to their nursing carers, that is, physical concerns and withheld others, for example, those relating to impact on daily life and fears for the future or of becoming a burden. This was despite the fact that the nurses considered themselves to be providing holistic care and had undertaken basic skills training. It must be noted however that in a recent study (Anderson *et al.* 2001) it was reported that patients disclosed over 90 per cent of troublesome concerns, although some differences were found between disclosure of physical, psychological, and social concerns.

Patients' fears

Patients fear being open about their situations and concerns (Peters-Golden 1982; Heaven and Maguire 1998). Many fear the stigma of cancer, especially the elderly for whom cancer equates with death (Maguire 1985), those whose lifestyles could have contributed to the illness, for example smokers, or those who come from a culture where cancer is less openly accepted (Parker and Hopwood 2000).

Stockwell (1972) studied the behaviour of nurses and identified that patients who were less jovial, depressed, or had many concerns and demands were unpopular and received less attention than those who were high spirited, fun, and easy to care for. Patients like to be liked and fear saying or doing anything that will make them unpopular with the staff. Patients fear burdening the staff with their many worries, allowing staff to see that they are not coping, or talking to staff about difficulties with side-effects, in case they are seen to be ungrateful, or worse still in case treatment is stopped (Maguire *et al.* 1980).

Other patients fear that if they talk about their concerns they will not be able to maintain composure and may risk breaking down and crying. Patients worry about burdening those around them and thus become highly protective of others, for fear of causing distress. This is well documented in terms of protection or withholding from relatives (Pistrang and Barker 1992) but is less often discussed in relation to protection of the professional carers. Insights into this phenomena were gained from the hospice study (Heaven and Maguire 1997), when a patient who told two nurses completely different concerns was interviewed. The patient said

> 'The first nurse was so sweet and nice, I did not want to hurt her by telling her all about that. Nurse 'X' on the other hand seemed stronger, less fragile, I felt I could tell her all my troubles.'

This response raises important issues for palliative care. The line between being a personal and professional friend should always be kept clear, lest the patient starts to protect the professional and closes off to themselves a line of support.

Patients' attitudes and beliefs

Patients hold beliefs that are not necessarily accurate or helpful in the quest for open communication. Many believe that certain problems are an inevitable part of having cancer and that health professionals would automatically recognize the presence of such difficulties and would offer help if available. They assume that lack of help being offered must mean that the problem cannot be alleviated and do not want to embarrass nurses and doctors by asking for the impossible (Rosser and Maguire 1982; Maguire 1985; Heaven and Maguire 1997).

Patients also believe that there is not enough time to go into all their worries. They therefore prioritize worries on the basis of what they think the professional will need or want to hear about, quite wrongly believing that certain types of professionals are only interested in certain types of problems or concerns (Heaven and Maguire 1997). A palliative care doctor may thus be told about issues such as physical symptoms and treatments, whilst a nurse may be told about issues such as deficits in self-care and the family situation.

Other patient factors

The final category of factors that affects patient disclosure is the physical factors. These include a lack of privacy from people, especially in a ward environment or a lack of space away from key individuals in front of whom that patient or relative may not wish to discuss certain fears (for example, spouses or children. Many health professionals do not consider the impact of the presence of a family member on an interview. In palliative care, professionals positively encourage the carer to be present when interviewing the patient; however, this may lead to many concerns being withheld, as patients actively protect their relatives (Pistrang and Barker 1992).

For many patients finding the right words is another difficulty that inhibits their ability to disclose concerns (Maguire 1985). Some individuals have a broad and extensive vocabulary for describing emotions but some will never have talked about their emotions. They may simply not have the words to describe how they feel or what they are experiencing. This is particularly relevant for certain groups, for example, those who are conducting the interview in a language that is not their first or native tongue or those who are mentally impaired due to illness (Morita *et al.* 2001) or learning difficulties. The danger for health professionals is that they may jump to the wrong conclusion, by filling in too many gaps or by not providing sufficient time and space.

Summary

The literature reveals a great number of reasons why communication difficulties occur. To date no study has compared the relative impact of the different influences identified and therefore there is no way of knowing which represents the greatest influence on behaviour. Indeed it is probable that the influence is different for each individual. There are many valid reasons why healthcare professionals may be ill at ease in talking openly and frankly to patients and why patients or relatives may withhold so much information about their fears and concerns.

Step 2: developing effective interviewing

What are effective interviewing skills?

The evidence for what constitutes an effective interview style has been developed over a number of years. This review will draw on literature that has researched the effectiveness of medical student, GP, nursing, psychotherapy, and psychiatry interviews. In 1979, Marks *et al.* conducted a study with GPs and showed that a number of key skills were associated with better interview outcomes, that is, more accurate identification of psychological morbidity. Key skills were

- using more eye contact at the outset of an interview
- clarifying more about the presenting complaint
- responding to verbal cues about possible distress
- asking directly about feelings
- asking about the home situation
- handling interruptions well
- making supportive comments.

This study was replicated by Goldberg *et al.* (1980) in the USA; Goldberg added to the list of facilitative behaviours:

- using directive questions about specific problems and using open questions more generally
- coping with talkativeness
- responding to verbal and non-verbal cues
- showing empathy.

The group also showed that reading notes while the patient talks is inhibitory. Studies suggested that changes in question style seem appropriate when seeking specific information about a specific issue or when establishing what the issues and events had been. Responding to patient cues was important but the only non-verbal behaviour identified as having an impact on outcome was eye contact. The importance of eye contact and responding to cues was further supported by a study by Davenport *et al.* (1987) who found that verbal cues were a better predictor of emotional distress.

Support for a more proactive enquiring style of interviewing was given by a Dutch group (Bensing and Sluijs 1985). They evaluated the effectiveness of teaching GPs a more passive style of interviewing, but patients gave a more confused history of events and disclosed significantly fewer of their key problems. These results are backed up by an US study (Putnam *et al.* 1988), which confirmed that teaching medical residents a more passive interview style showed no improvement in clinical outcomes.

Integrating physical and psychological modes of enquiry was found to be very important by Cox *et al.* (1988). They compared a traditional medical interview style with a more integrated style, where the interviewers sought detailed information about changes in behaviour and symptoms, but also the feelings these had generated. The latter style significantly improved disclosure of the quality and quantity of factual information and associated feelings.

So the evidence supports the view that to be effective an interview must include detailed probing about key events and requests for the associated feelings, clarification of both verbal and non-verbal cues particularly about distress, establishment and maintainence of good eye contact, and enquiry about the impact of any key problems on the patient's functioning, psychological adjustment, and home situation.

Most of this evidence however has come from general practice and medical training situations. The relevance of these skills to other professional groups and to the cancer or palliative care situation was the focus of a study by Maguire *et al.* (1996). Earlier work (Maguire *et al.* 1980) had shown that nurses trained to ask open questions about feelings and respond to cues empathetically were more effective in establishing patients' emotional concerns and concerns about side-effects. The 1996 study set out to validate the model of communication being taught in a multi-professional context (Maguire and Faulkner 1988) and involved the assessment of interviews conducted by 206 healthcare professionals. Results showed that disclosure of key information, emotions, and concerns was significantly affected by the skills shown and defined as follows:

Facilitative behaviours

These include

(1) open directive questions—questions which give a broad focus but are open, for example, 'How have you been since I last saw you?';

(2) questions with a psychological focus—eliciting information about emotions, worries, concerns, and fears;

(3) clarification of psychological aspects—any behaviour that seeks to understand more about any emotional aspect;

(4) empathy—a brief statement showing understanding of the patient's experience;

(5) summarizing—a recapitulation of two or more items previously discussed;

(6) educated guesses—an educated guess is a tentative behaviour in which the interviewer makes a guess or hypothesis about the situation, based upon feelings or 'gut reactions' with the patient, and then allows the patient to respond to confirm or refute it.

Inhibitory behaviours

These include

(1) leading questions—questions that suggest or presuppose the answer;

(2) physically focused questions—questions that limit the topic to the physical experience of the patient;

(3) clarifying the physical aspects—any behaviour that seeks to understand more about the physical experience of the patient;

(4) giving of any advice—any information given to the patient before or after exploration of the concerns.

A ratio of one facilitative to every three inhibitory behaviours was noted by Maguire *et al.* (1996) regardless of the interviewer's age, experience, or professional grouping.

Summary

To be effective, an interviewer needs to be proactive and use open and directive questions to elicit patients' experiences (for example, 'How is chemotherapy going?') and then acknowledge and clarify cues given about important problems and distress. The use of empathy and educated questions is likely to encourage patients to disclose associated feelings. Repeated summarizing of what the interviewer has heard lets patients know that they have been understood correctly or allows them to correct the interviewer. The establishment and maintenance of good eye contact is key. The integration of enquiry about physical symptoms, psychological impact, social impact, and effect of spirituality is particularly important.

What are effective information-giving skills?

So far effective interviewing has only been considered in terms of assessment. The process of giving information, specifically bad news is now considered. The importance of the bad-news interview on patient adjustment has been shown (Butow *et al.* 1996), however very little research has been conducted that identifies how aspects of the process affect patient outcome.

Mager and Andrykowski (2002) established that long-term distress was related to the 'caring skills', that is, the empathy and responsiveness, of the doctor and not their technical competence. Fallowfield *et al.* (1990) showed that adjustment was related to meeting patients' information needs appropriately. Too much or too little information can be detrimental to a patient's mental health (Fallowfield *et al.* 1990), indicating that the amount of information given should be tailored to need and that the pace of delivery should be dictated by the recipient (Maguire 1998). There is also evidence that using audiorecordings can assist patients in taking on board complex information (Hogbin *et al.* 1992) but that they may be detrimental if the news received is of a poor prognosis (McHugh *et al.* 1995). Cultural background has not been found to affect a patients desire to know about their diagnosis (Fielding and Hunt 1996; Seo *et al.* 2000), although relatives have a greater influence in some cultures than in others (Mosoiu *et al.* 2000; Di Mola and Crisci 2001).

Girghis and Sanson-Fisher (1995) created guidelines on breaking bad news that were drawn up on the basis of a comprehensive literature review and recommendations from doctors and cancer patients. The guidelines covered practical issues, such as privacy and adequate time, and strategy of approach, such as assessing the patient's current understanding, providing information simply and honestly, being realistic concerning time-frames and prognosis, avoiding euphemisms, encouraging patients to express feelings, and being empathic. Miller and Maguire (2000) drew similar conclusions from a systematic review of the literature, however they found some evidence that using euphemisms to deliver bad news in a step-wise fashion was beneficial for patients who are totally unaware of diagnoses.

The longitudinal study conducted by Parle *et al.* (1996) suggested that a key element in bad-news consultation was to acknowledge the distress the bad news had created and then invite the patient to explain proactively how they were feeling and the concerns that were contributing to that distress. The patient should then be invited to prioritize their concerns so that each concern can be taken in order. Only then should further information be given, based on what information patients want at that point.

This approach has been the subject of a randomized trial being conducted by the Cancer Research UK Psychological Medicine Group in Manchester. The preliminary data suggest that this model not only increases the chances that patients will disclose their concerns but also reduces their distress. Moreover, it helps the doctors feel better about the way they are breaking bad news and gives them validation that they are helping rather than upsetting patients.

Summary

Whilst it is clear that the process of giving bad news is crucial to long-term adjustment, little evidence exists as to what constitutes effective practice. It is clear that information must be tailored to individual needs no matter what culture the individual comes from and that it should be given in 'bite-sized chunks' at a pace that is controlled by the patient. Empathy and understanding is crucial.

Acquiring effective interviewing skills

So far only the types of skills that are required have been discussed. The question of how these skills may be acquired is now considered. There have been a number of published studies on communication skills training, however, few of the communication skills training programmes available have been evaluated formally to assess their effectiveness in achieving desired outcomes. This section, therefore, considers the key elements of effective communication skills training, so that individuals can assess the value of potential courses.

Early studies conducted with medical students measured outcomes in terms of changes in interviewing behaviour and ability to identify diagnoses and problems. These experimental studies showed the value in a didactic introduction to a model of interviewing behaviour together with some kind of demonstration of that model working in practice (Rutter and Maguire 1976; Maguire *et al.* 1977). Subsequent evidence confirmed the value of feedback on individual performance as being essential, with video and audio feedback conferring equal benefit (Maguire *et al.* 1978). An alternative training approach developed in the USA and shown to be effective in nurse and doctor training, is micro-counselling training (Daniels *et al.* 1988; Crute *et al.* 1989). This uses the same core elements of training but focuses on one micro-skill per session, rather than one strategy or task, as described in the studies already mentioned.

Studies of the problems of open and honest communication highlighted the important role of attitudes and beliefs (Wilkinson 1991; Booth *et al.* 1996). This led to training that focused on attitudes; but a comparison study showed that attitude training alone was not sufficient to change communication behaviour and that training had to encompass a skills focus if skills were to be changed (Rickert 1982).

The role of attitudes however must not be overlooked, as was shown by Razavi *et al.* (1988) and by Maguire *et al.* (1996). The 1996 UK-based evaluation showed that the training conferred many positive skill changes in communication skills but did not confer changes in the key skills of empathy and educated guesses. Furthermore it was found that whilst training that addresses skills alone leads to more significant and emotional disclosure from the patient, it also leads to significantly more blocking on the part of the professional.

To overcome these difficulties, changes were implemented so that workshops provided more time for practising skills and for feedback on performance and greater safety to address attitudes, beliefs, and fears about possible consequences of the communication process. The structural issues of interviewing, for example, learning about how long to remain with one particular topic, when and how to move on, as well as how to integrate the factual, physical, and emotional modes of interviewing were explored. The experimental evaluation showed that the optimal training method was one that addressed not only skills but also interview structure and professionals' attitudes and feelings. This multi-dimensional focus in training has now been shown to be highly effective in different contexts (Razavi et al. 2000; Heaven 2001; Fallowfield et al. 2002).

Summary

For communication skills training to be effective there appear to be key elements that need to be in place. These include presentation of a clear, evidence-based model of communication, demonstration of that model, opportunity for trainees to practise skills in a safe environment, and explicit but constructive feedback on performance. Furthermore, to be effective training needs not only to take account of skills but also to challenge beliefs and overcome fears and it needs to teach integration of factual, physical, emotional, spiritual, and social domains.

Step 3: transferring skills to the workplace and maintaining them over time

The final step to changing communication behaviour is to ensure transfer of learning to the work place and to maintain improvement in skills over time. There appears to be a difference between what a health professional can do in interviewing simulated patients and what they actually do when faced with real patients or relatives. Parle et al. (1997) suggested that this difference could be accounted for by Bandura's learning theory. They highlighted the importance of considering self-efficacy, a person's confidence in their ability to perform a communication task successfully and outcome expectancy, a personal belief that the outcome of using a specific skill or strategy will benefit both themselves and their patient.

Within the communication skills training literature, 'drop-off' in skills has been noted (Maguire et al. 1996; Wilkinson et al. 1998) as has the inability of trainees to apply skills in a clinically meaningful way (Putman et al. 1988; Heaven and Maguire 1996; Razavi et al. 1990). A much greater understanding of the problem of transfer can be gained from other applied psychology literature, where the phenomena has been researched in great depth (Gist et al. 1990). In a major literature review, Baldwin and Ford (1988) point to a number of key factors in facilitating transfer: first, before training there needs to be real commitment not only to learning but also to behaviour change, second, the training has to be effective, and finally the environment into which the trainee is returning must be supportive. There is strong evidence to support the notion that for skills to be effectively transferred back into the workplace, both general support and more specifically facilitated integration of skills appear to be crucial (Gist *et al.* 1990; Bandura 1992).

These factors have been the focus of the authors' most recent work, in which the role of clinical supervision in effecting transfer of communication skills training from workshop to workplace was investigated. Sixty-one clinical nurse specialists (70% of whom were palliative 'care nurses) participated in a randomized, controlled trial of workshop training alone compared with workshop training plus a four-week integration programme using clinical supervision (Heaven 2001). Those nurses who had received supervision used significantly more facilitative communication skills with patients and relatives, responded to cues in a more facilitative fashion, and were more able to identify concerns of an emotional nature, than those who had not.

If the key to transfer is facilitating the integration of skills into practice, it is logical to assume that programmes of training that extend over a period of time will be more effective. Wilkinson *et al.* (1998) published a study of nurses who had undergone a programme of communication skills training as part of a palliative care course (Wilkinson *et al.* 1998). The results showed significant improvements in the nurses' interviewing behaviours with real patients over the course of the training programme, suggesting that this method of training may overcome the transfer problem. Wilkinson *et al.* (2001), however, compared workshop training with an integrated programme of training. They found both conferred equal learning and transfer, suggesting that the apparent transfer effect could be due to other factors. The use of intensive workshop training, following a similar format to that previously discussed, has been shown to have a clinically measurable effect, which was transferred back into the workplace by the senior doctors undergoing the training (Fallowfield *et al.* 2002). This training was highly intensive (one facilitator, four participants) and provided written feedback on performance for a randomized sample of participants. Written feedback was not found to confer greater learning or use of skills.

The conclusion of the studies is that transfer of skills to the workplace must not be assumed. To ensure integration of skills and facilitate maintenance over time, support within the workplace and help during the integration process is key. Extended or highly intensive training may overcome some of these problems, as may workplace structures such as clinical supervision (Heaven 2001).

The key objective of any intervention aimed at facilitating transfer should be to provide a forum in which self-efficacy can be boosted, negative outcome expectancies challenged, and emotional and practical support provided (Bandura 1992; Gist *et al.* 1990; Heaven 2001). Other methods include informal peer supervision, in which two or three individuals meet together with the purpose of discussing specific difficulties. Alternatively, individual reflection or a personal de-briefing or encounter (Newell 1992) can provide a forum in which the individual can challenge their assumptions, attribution, purpose, and outcomes and gain confidence in their abilities and outcomes.

Support for skills can be elicited during the course of a normal day through feedback from the patient, 'chats' with colleagues about specific events, and team meetings at which views can be validated and ideas endorsed. There is evidence that many people leave courses with good intentions about using skills but often these are not put into practice. Goal setting may help avoid this, as may reviewing courses after a period of time, to appraise how much trainees feel they have used the skills learned (Bird *et al.* 1993; Baile *et al.* 1997; Fallowfield *et al.* 1998). Another method of self-appraisal is audiorecording an interview, with the patient's full consent, and then reviewing it. It is important to remember that to boost self-efficacy positive reinforcement is very important, therefore a balanced appraisal is critical. The final method available to maintain learning is to regularly reappraise learning needs and further training courses that offer the chance to re-look at skills or to learn new skills (Razavi *et al.* 1993). Initiatives in Scandinavia have shown that initial training followed by shorter booster workshops have been very effective in changing practice, when evaluated subjectively (Aspegren *et al.* 1996).

The key to transfer appears to be recognizing that intentions and actions are not the same, and that without specific action and support, changes in competence are not necessarily translated into changes in performance.

References

Anderson H, Ward C, Eardley A, Gomm S, Connolly M, Coppinger T *et al.* (2001). The concerns of patients under palliative care and a heart failure clinic are not being met. *Palliative Med* 15:279–86.

Ashcroft JJ, Leinster SJ, Slade PD (1985). Breast cancer—patient choice of treatment: preliminary communication *J R Soc Med* 78:43–6.

Aspegren K, Birgegard G, Ekeberg O, Hietanen P, Holm U, Jensen AB (1996). Improving awareness of the psychosocial needs of the paient—a training course for experienced cancer doctors. *Acta Oncol* 35:246–8.

Baider L, Porath S (1981). Uncovering fear: group experience of nurses in a cancer ward. *Int J Nursing Stud* 18:47–52.

Baile W, Lenzi R, Kudelka A, Maguire P, Novack D, Goldstein M *et al.* (1997). Improving physician–patient communication in cancer care: outcome of a workshop for oncologists. *J Cancer Ed* 12:66–173.

Baldwin TT, Ford JK (1988). Transfer of training: a review and directions for future research. *Personnel Psychol* 41:63–105.

Bandura A. (1977). Self-efficacy: toward a unifying theory of behavioral change. *Psychol Rev* 84:191–215.

Bandura A. (1992). Psychological aspects of prognostic judgements. In: Evans, Baskin, Yatsu (ed.). *Prognosis of neurological disorders*. pp. 13–28.

Bensing JM, Sluijs EM (1985). Evaluation of an interview training course for general practitioners. *Soc Sci Med* 20:737–44.

Bird J, Hall A, Heavy A (1993). Workshops for consultants on the teaching of clinical communication skills. *Med Ed* 27:181–5.

Bond S (1983). Nurses' communication with cancer patients. In: Wilson-Barnett J (ed.). *Ten studies in patient care*. John Wiley & Sons.

Booth K, Maguire P, Butterworth T, Hillier VF (1996). Perceived professional support and the use of blocking behaviours by hospice nurses. *J Adv Nursing* 24:522–7.

Bornstein B, Emler C (2001). Rationality in medical decision making: a review of the literature on doctors decision-making biases. *J Eval Clin Pract* 7:97–107.

Bredin M, Corner J, Krishnasamy M, Plant H, Bailey C, A'Hearn R (1999). Multicentre randomised controlled trial of nursing intervention for breathlessness in patients with lung cancer. *BMJ* 318:901–4.

Brown I (1981). The effects of a death education programme for nurses working in a long-term care hospital. *Diss Abstr Int* 42:54A.

Butow PN, Kazemi J, Beeney L, Griffin A, Dunn S, Tattersall M (1996). When the diagnosis is cancer: patient communication experiences and preferences. *Cancer* 77:2630–7.

Cheturvedi S, Shenoy A, Prasad K, Senthilnathan S, Premlatha B (1996). Concerns, coping and quality of life in head and neck cancer patients *Support Care Cancer* 4:186–90.

Coulter A (1999). Paternalism or partnership? Patients have grown-up and there's no going back. *BMJ* 319:719–20.

Cox A, Rutter M, Holbrook D (1988). Psychiatric interviewing: a second experimental study: eliciting feelings. *Br J Psychiat* 152:64–72.

Cox K (2002). Informed consent and decision-making: patients' experiences of the process of recruitment to phase I and II anti-cancer drug trials. *Patient Ed Counseling* 46:31–8.

Crow R, Chase J, Lamond D (1995). The cognitive component of nursing assessment: an analysis. *Journal of Advanced Nursing* 22(2):206–12.

Crute VC, Hargie ODW, Ellis RAF (1989). An evaluation of a communication skills course for health visitor students. *J AdvNursing,* 14:546–52.

Daniels TG, Denny A, Andrews D (1988). Using microcounseling to teach RN students skills of therapeutic communication. *J Nursing Ed* 27:246–52.

Davenport S, Goldberg D, Miller T (1987). How psychiatric disorders are missed during medical consultations. *Lancet* 4:439–41.

de Valch C, Bensing J, Bruynooghe R (2001). Medical students' attitudes towards breaking bad news: an emperical test of the world health organisation model. *Psycho-oncology* 10:398–409.

Delvaux N, Razavi D, Farvaques C (1988). Cancer care—a stress for health professionals. *Soc Sci Med* 27:159–66.

Derogatis LR, Morrow GR, Fetting J, Penman D, Piasetsky S, Schmale AM *et al.* (1983). The prevalence of psychiatric disorders among cancer patients. *JAMA* 249:751–7.

DiMola G, Crisci M (2001). Attitudes towards death and dying in a representative sample of the Italian population. *Palliative Med* 15:372–8.

Dowsett SM, Saul JL, Butow PN, Dunn SM, Boyer MJ, Findlow R *et al.* (2000). Communication style in the cancer consultation: preferences for a pateint-centred approach. *Psycho-oncology* 9:147–56.

Duldt BW (1982). Helping nurses to cope with the anger-dismay syndrome. *Nursing Outlook* March:168–74.

Fallowfield L, Lipkin M, Hall A (1998). Teaching senior oncologists communication skills: results from phase 1 of a comprehensive longitudinal program in the United Kingdom. *J Clin Oncol* 16:1961–8.

Fallowfield LJ, Hall A, Maguire P, Baum M (1990). Psychological outcomes of different treatment policies in women with early breast cancer outside a clinical trial *BMJ* 301:575–80.

Fallowfield L, Jenkins V, Farewell V, Saul J, Duffy A, Eves R (2002). Efficacy of a cancer research UK communication skills training model for oncologists: a randomised controlled trial. *Lancet* **359**:650–6.

Field D, Kitson C (1986). Formal teaching about dealth and dying in UK nursing schools. *Nurse Ed Today* **6**:270–6.

Fielding R, Hunt J (1996). Preferences for information and involvement in decisions during cancer care among a Hong Kong Chinese population. *Psycho-oncology* **5**:321–9.

Fielding RG, Llewelyn SP (1987). Communication training in nursing may damage your health and enthusiasm: some warnings. *Journal of Advanced Nursing* **12**:281–90.

Ford S, Fallowfield L, Lewis S (1996). Doctor–patient interactions in oncology. *Soc Sci Med* **42**:1511–19.

Fulton C (1998). The prevalence and detection of psychiatric morbidity in patients with metastatic breast cancer. *Eur J Cancer Care* **7**:232–9.

Girghis A, Sanson-Fisher R (1995). Breaking bad news: consensus guidelines for medical practitioners. *J Clin Oncol* **13**:2449–56.

Gist ME, Bavettw AG, Stevens CK (1990). Transfer training method: its influence on skill generalization, skill repetition, and skill performance level. *Personnel Psychol* **43**:501–23.

Glajchen M, Blum D, Calder K (1995). Cancer pain management and the role of social work: barriers and interventions. *Health Soc Work* **20**:200–6.

Goldberg DP, Steele JJ, Smith C, Spivey L (1980). Training the family doctors to recognise psychiatric illness with increased accuracy. *Lancet* **September**:521–3.

Grey-Toft P, Anderson JG (1981). Stress among hospital nursing staff: its causes and effects. *Soc Sci Med* **15A**:639–47.

Hanson EJ (1994). An exploration of the taken-for-granted world of the cancer nurse in relation to stress and the person with cancer. *Journal of Advanced Nursing* **19**:12–20.

Hardman A, Maguire P, Crowther D (1989). The recognition of psychiatric morbidity on a medical oncology ward. *J Psychosomat Res* **33**:235–9.

Heaven CM (2001). The role of clinical supervision in communication skills training [PhD Thesis]. Manchester: University of Manchester.

Heaven CM, Maguire P (1996). Training hospice nurses to elicit patient concerns. *J Adv Nursing* **23**:280–6.

Heaven CM, Maguire P (1997). Disclosure of concerns by hospice patients and their identification by nurses. *Palliative Med* **11**:283–90.

Heaven CM, Maguire P (1998). The relationship between patients' concerns and psychological distress in hospice setting. *Psycho-oncology* **7**:502–7.

Hinds C, Streter A, Mood D (1995). Functions and preferred methods of receiving information related to radiotherapy. Perceptions of patients wth cancer. *Cancer Nurse* **18**:374–84.

Hitch PJ, Murgatroyd JD (1983). Professional communications in cancer care: a Delphi survey of hospital nurses. *J Adv Nursing* **8**:413–422.

Hobgin B, Jenkins VA, Parkin AJ (1992). Remembering 'bad news' consultations: an evaluation of tape-recorded consultations. *Psycho-oncology* **1**:147–54.

Huckaby L, Neal M (1979). The nursing care plan problem. *J Nursing Admin* **9**:36–42.

Ibbotson T, Maguire P, Selby P, Priestman T, Wallace L (1994). Screening for anxiety and depresson in cancer patients: the effects of disease and treatment. *Eur J Cancer* **30A**:37–40.

Kai-Hoi Sze F, Wong E, Lo R, Woo J (2000). Do pain and disability differ in depressed cancer patients. *Palliative Med* 14:11–17.

Kissane D, Bloch S, Burns WI, McKenzie DP, Posterino M (1994). Psychological morbidity in the families of patients with cancer. *Psycho-oncology* 3:47–56.

Larson DG (1993). Self-concealment: implications for stress and empathy in oncology care. *Journal of Psychosocial Oncology* 11(4):1–16.

Lo R, Woo J, Zhoc K, Li C, Yeo W, Johnson P, Mak Y, Lee J (2001). Cross-cultural validation of the McGill quality of life questionnaire in Hong Kong Chinese. *Palliative Med* 15:387–97.

McElroy AM (1982). Burnout—a review of the literature with application to cancer nursing. *Cancer Nursing* June:211–17.

Macleod-Clark J (1983). Nurse-patient communication—an analysis of conversations from surgical wards in Nursing research. In: Wilson-Barnett J (ed.). *Ten studies in patient care.* John Wiley & Sons.

Mager W, Andrykowski M (2002). Communication in the cancer 'bad news' consultation: patient perceptions and psychological adjustment. *Psycho-oncology* 11:11–46.

Maguire P (1985). Improving the detection of psychiatric problems in cancer patients. *SocSci Med* 20:819–23.

Maguire P (1998). Breaking bad news. *Eur J Surg Oncol* 24:188–91.

Maguire P (1999). Improving communication with cancer patients. *Eur J Cancer* 35:1415–22.

Maguire P, Faulkner A (1988). Improving the counselling skills of doctors and nurses in cancer care. *BMJ* 297:847–9.

Maguire GP, Clarke D, Jolley B (1977). An experimental comparison of three courses in history-taking skills for medical students. *Med Ed* 11:175–82.

Maguire P, Roe P, Goldberg D, Jones S, Hyde C, O'Dowd T (1978). The value of feedback in teaching interviewing skills to medical students. *Psychol Med* 8:695–704.

Maguire P, Tait A, Brooke M, Thomas C, Sellwood R (1980). Effect of counselling on the psychiatric morbidity assiciated with mastectomy. *BMJ* 281:1454–6.

Maguire P, Faulkner A, Booth K, Elliot C, Hillier V (1996). Helping cancer patients disclose their concerns. *Eur J Cancer* 32A:78–81.

Marks JN, Goldberg DP, Hillier VF (1979). Determinants of the ability of general practitioners to detect psychiatric illness. *Psychol Med* 9:337–53.

McHugh P, Lewis S, Ford S, Newlands E, Rustin G, Coombes C *et al* (1995). The efficacy of audiotapes in promoting psychological well-being in cancer patients: a randomised controlled trial. *Br J Cancer* 71:388–92.

Miller S, Maguire P (2000). Breaking bad news to adult cancer patients: a review of the evidence [personal communication].

Moorhead R, Winefield H (1991). Teaching counselling skills to fourth-year medical students: a dilemma concerning goals. *Family Pract* 8:343–6.

Morita T, Tsunoda J, Inoue S, Chihara S, Oka K (2001). Communication capacity scale and agitation dsitress scale to measure the severity of delirium in terminally ill cancer patients: a validation study. *Palliative Med* 15:197–206.

Morris J, Royle GT (1987). Choice of surgery for early breast cancer: pre and post operative levels of clinical anxiety and depression in patients and their husbands. *BrJ Surg* 74:1017–19.

Mosoiu D, Andrews C, Perolls G (2000). Palliative care in Romania. *Palliative Med* 14:65–7.

Newell R (1992). Anxiety, accuracy and reflection: the limits of professional development. *J Adv Nursing,* **17**:1326–33.

Parker R, Hopwood P (2000). Literature review—quality of life (QL) in black and ethnic monority groups (BEMGs) with cancer. CRC Report. London: Cancer Research UK.

Parle M, Jones B, Maguire P (1996). Maladaptive coping and affective disorders in cancer patients. *Psychol Med* **26**:735–44.

Parle M, Maguire P, Heaven CM (1997). The development of a training model to improve health profesionals' skills, self-efficacy and outcome expectancies when communicating with cancer patients. *Soc Sci Med* **44**:231–40.

Peters-Golden H (1982). Breast cancer, varied perception of social support in the illness experience. *Soc Sci Med* **16**:483–91.

Peterson M (1988). The norms and values held by three groups of nurses concerning psychosocial nursing practice. *Int J Nursing Stud* **25**:85–103.

Pistrang N, Barker C (1992). Disclosure of concerns in breast cancer. *Psycho-oncology* **1**:183–92.

Pitceathly P, Maguire P (2000). Preventing affective disorders in partners of cancer patients; an intervention study. In: Baider L, Cooper CL, Kaplan De-Nour AK (ed.). *Cancer and the family.* pp. 137–54.

Putnam S.M, Stiles WB, Jacob MC, James SA (1988). Teaching the medical interview: an intervention study. *J Gen Intern Med* **3**:38–47.

Ramirez AJ, Graham J, Richards MA, Cull A, Gregory W.M (1996). Mental health of hospital consultants: the effects of stress and satifaction at work. *Lancet* **347**:724–8.

Razavi D, Delvaux N, Farvaques C, Robaye E (1988). Immediate effectiveness of brief psychological training for health professionals dealing with terminally ill cancer patients: a controlled study. *Social Science and Medicine* **27**(4):369–75.

Razavi D, Delvaux N, Farvacques C, Robaye E (1990). Screening for adjustment disorders and major depressive disorders in cancer in-patients. *Br J Psychiat* **156**:79–83.

Razavi D, Delvaux N, Marchal S, Bredart A, Farvacques C, Paesmans M (1993). The effects of a 24-h psychological training program on attitudes,communication skills and occupational stress in oncology: a randomised study. *Eur J Cancer* **29A**:1858–63.

Razavi D, Delvaux N, Marchal S, De Cock M, Farvaques C, Slachmuylder J-L (2000). Testing health care professionals' communication skills: the usefulness of highly emotional standardized role-playing sessions with simulators. *Psycho-oncology* **9**:293–302.

Richards M, Ramirez A, Degner L, Maher E, Neuberger J (1995). Offering choice to patients with cancers. A review based on a synposium held at the 10th annual conference of the British Psychosocial Oncology Group, December 1993. *Eur J Cancer* **31A**:112–16.

Rickert ML (1982). Terminal illness, dying and death: training for caregivers. *Diss Abstr Int* **42**:3443-A.

Rosser J, Maguire P (1982). Dilemmas in general practice: the care of the cancer patient. *Soc Sci Med* **16**:315–22.

Rothenbacher D, Lutz M, Porzsolt F (1997). Treatment decisions in palliative cancer care: Patients' preferences for involvement and doctors' knowledge about it. *EurJ Cancer* **33**:1184–9.

Rutter DR, Maguire GP (1976). History-taking for medical students. II—evaluation of a training programme. *Lancet* **September:** 558–60.

Sellick KJ (1991). Nurses' interpersonal behaviours and the development of helping skills. *Int J Nursing Stud* **28**:3–11.

Seo M, Tamura K, Shijo H, Morioka E, Ikegame C, Hirasako K (2000). Telling the diagnosis to cancer patients in Japan: attitude and perception of patients, physicians and nurses. *Palliative Med* **14**:105–10.

Smith M, Hart G (1994). Nurses' responses to patient anger: from disconnecting to connecting. *Journal of Advanced Nursing* **20**:643–51.

Stockwell F (1972). *The unpopular patient.* London: Royal College of Nursing.

Tait A (1994). Breast care nursing. London: Cancer Relief Macmillan Fund.

Weisman AD, Worden JW (1977). The existential plight of cancer: significance of the first 100 days. *IntJ Psychol Med* **7**:1–15.

Wilkinson S (1991). Factors which influence how nurses communicate with cancer patients. *J Adv Nursing* **16**:677–88.

Wilkinson S, Roberts A, Aldridge J (1998). Nurse–patient communication in palliative care; an evaluation of a communication skills programme. *Palliative Med* **12**:13–22.

Wilkinson S, Leliopoulou C, Gambles M, Roberts A (2001). The long and short of it: a comparison of outcomes of two approaches to teaching communication skills. In: *Seventeenth Annual Scientific Meeting of the British Psychosocial Oncology Society*, London.

Chapter 3

Social impact of advanced metastatic cancer

Frances Sheldon

Introduction

From the moment that someone learns that there is no further curative treatment for their advancing metastatic cancer that person sees themselves differently and is perceived differently by those around them. How differently depends on the meaning attributed to the news and the coping styles of those individuals. One person may see this as a challenge to a fight that they are still determined to win, another as a death sentence, to which they can only respond with sadness and withdrawal. Those around the dying person may subscribe to that person's approach or see the situation quite differently. So understanding what may be involved as both the dying person and those connected with them struggle with a changing identity is crucial in working with those experiencing the social impact of advanced cancer. Of course not every dying person or every family member is specifically told of the situation, but the physical and possibly also mental deterioration experienced necessarily changes relationships and function in the short or long term. This developing awareness may occur early in the trajectory of the illness or after many years of relapse, treatment, and remission.

That there is social pain alongside physical, psychological, and spiritual pain has long been recognized in palliative care but it is probably the least-understood aspect of 'total pain' (Field 2000). This chapter aims to change that and to explore in more detail some of the components of social pain (Plate 2, pp. 98–99). We will first consider some of the broad issues relating to identity at this time, to dependence and independence, in the light of different contexts and different cultural backgrounds. Then we will look more specifically at the impact of advanced cancer on family relationships and the dying person's social situation and ways in which professional interventions and service provision may support those involved and ameliorate that impact.

Social contexts for death and bereavement

Our identity is developed in a social context over our lifespan, though, as Lawton (2000) indicates in her research study of the bodily realities of dying, this is also inextricably bound up with our inner sense of being. The social context in which death and bereavement take place is changing. Walter (1994) has charted three types of context for dying. The first is the traditional context where death occurs in a community setting with close involvement of family and friends and where religion often provides the framework that offers both meaning and ritual. The second is the modern context where the authority of medicine is paramount, the hospital is the predominant setting, and emotion and information are kept private and controlled, both by family members and by staff caring for the dying person. The third is a neo-modern approach where the dying person is much more self-determining. There is again more openness about what is happening, as in the traditional context. The dying person may even write about their emotions and experiences in a regular newspaper column, seek to control where death occurs, and plan the funeral.

As Walter (1994) points out, in a country like the UK all these three contexts may be operating. The traditional context may be found in some rural or migrant communities. The neo-modern approach is probably more often found among younger people (John Diamond and Ruth Picardie are well-known examples) than among older people who grew up through the middle of the twentieth century when medical and other types of authority were more highly respected. Families too develop their own individual cultures in response to the family history, the society in which they live, and the balancing of the contributions of the different members. So a particular family may wish to operate in neo-modern mode even when living in a traditional society.

In addition to the societal context and the familial culture, the cultural history and current cultural orientation of both the dying person and their family play a significant part in shaping the social impact of advancing cancer. As so many writers on cultural aspects of palliative care have observed, 'cultures are dynamic and not homogeneous' (Firth 2001). So knowing that someone emigrated from the west of Ireland as a young man forty years ago may provide useful background information but only a respectful and sensitive exploration of his present attitudes and beliefs will determine how influential those current in his childhood still are for him (Donnelly 1999). Firth (1997) reports that many hospitals in India send those that are dying back home because of the importance in Hindu culture of dying at home, well prepared and surrounded by a particular set of rituals. A younger generation of Hindus born in the UK may have very different expectations from their parents who were born in India and there may in any case be no qualified priest available to perform the rituals, so lay members of the community may need to substitute.

Culture links to the spiritual aspects of life, which are dealt with elsewhere in this book, and these too will influence the impact of advancing cancer on social relationships. In the Jewish faith it is important to maintain hope (Neuberger 1993). This may mean that openness about a terminal prognosis with the patient may not be acceptable to a Jewish family, with the consequences that may bring for resolution of unfinished business or acceptance of support from a Macmillan nurse. Culture similarly influences decision making in families and perceptions of dependence and independence. The anxiety about 'being a burden' and loss of autonomy, so evident in Western societies (Seale and Addington-Hall 1994), is less weighty in cultures where older people are more valued, where parents are still the decision makers in the family even when old, and where the family rather than the individual is significant.

Finally, gender is a factor to be considered in how the dying person and those involved with that person respond to advancing cancer. It has been most explored in bereavement where research by Stroebe (1998) indicates that on the whole men in Western societies are more problem focused and women more emotion focused in their reactions. Although it has not so far been specifically researched in relation to men or women caring for dying people, it does appear from the literature on caring in general that men carers (the minority) are more task oriented and adopt a more 'formal' approach than women carers, for whom a sense of duty and the expectation that it is part of a woman's identity are still significant (Neale 1991). Interestingly Lawton (2000) observes that for the seriously ill patients in the hospice she studied, gender differences in response to their illness were not marked. The bodily deterioration that these men and women had experienced had made them feel that they had lost much of what made them 'masculine' or 'feminine'. However professionals working with dying people and those involved with them need to be clear about all the particular influences from their social and cultural contexts if they are to offer appropriate care.

The nature of social pain

Employment and income

The losses experienced by people with advanced cancer in relation to their social world are concerned with their engagement with the world outside home and with the roles and relationships within the family. By the time the cancer is advanced many people of working age will have had to reduce or give up altogether their engagement in employment. For some this is the biggest loss and is resisted.

Bill, aged 45, was a scaffolding erector. His marriage had broken up and he had become homeless as a result of this and his difficulty in earning because of his brain tumour which was producing frequent dizzy spells. He had a new girlfriend who was still married herself and living in the matrimonial home. Her husband was often away on business and had agreed that Bill could live in the cellar room of their house on a temporary basis. So much of his former identity had gone and he hated being dependent on the whim of his girlfriend's husband. So he tried at all costs to maintain his view of himself as a worker. When prospective clients called to book him he would tell them that he could not manage it this week but he would book them in next week. This considerably alarmed his girlfriend and the teams caring for him. They tried to confront him with the impossibility of clambering on roofs and up ladders but he brushed this aside. Over time it became clear that confrontation was not necessary because, although Bill remained in denial, he would always ring up and defer the client for yet another week when the booked date arrived. Thus he minimized the only aspect of his social pain that he felt he could control.

Financial hardship often goes hand in hand with serious illness. There may be additional expense for heat, food, and clothes at a time when income has stayed the same or reduced. For many this will be the first time in their lives they will have encountered the welfare benefits system or applied for charitable funds. Despite the efforts that have been made in the UK in recent years to simplify the language and layout of benefit application forms, they present a formidable challenge to a new user; for example, Jenny, caring for her bed-ridden husband and applying for 'attendance allowance' commented 'When they ask "Why do you want this help?" I don't know where to start.' But it is not just a practical issue. Stevenson (1973) has identified both the moral opprobrium that is often linked with poverty and the fact that being a claimant may also identify that person as someone who has 'failed' in some way. Particularly if you have always seen yourself as different from 'those layabouts on benefit who are given huge sums at the tax payer's expense', contemplating joining this group is extremely distressing. Similarly the symbolism of being a recipient of charity when you have always been a giver can prevent an application being made unless this issue is talked through first. It is interesting that this is an area often neglected by professionals (Sykes *et al.* 1992), perhaps because of fear of its sensitivity, though that does not stop detailed exploration of a patient's bowel habits! By acknowledging that this can be a problem, exploring what is most painful, not being too quick to reassure that somehow the ill person is different from other benefit or charity applicants (because in reality they are unlikely to be), but communicating that their worth and value are not changed, professionals can help claimants to tackle this step with less pain. Practical help in treading through the maze may well be needed alongside. Cancer and palliative care services can provide this, perhaps through a social worker, a volunteer who develops an expertise in this area, or through a link with the Citizens' Advice Bureau or local welfare benefits service.

Social engagement

As mobility and energies decline it becomes harder to participate in social events and maintain friendships that were built on sharing activities and interests. Social isolation is a frequent source of social pain for both the person with advanced cancer and any carers. Accessing local volunteer transport groups may help in maintaining old interests, if the loss of an ability to drive or use public transport is the problem. Even the provision of a disabled parking badge may make someone feel part of society again, through enabling common activities like shopping. Going on holiday is another valued social activity and charities like Macmillan Cancer Relief can provided support to make this possible. Hospice Information's booklet *Flying home—or on Holiday*, which gives advice about travel arrangements for very sick people, is a useful resource here, or for those who wish at a late stage to return to the country of their birth (Myers 2002).

For some, the change in the way they feel about themselves and their declining function create too big a gap between past social engagement and the present. For them a solution may be to participate in new social groups, such as cancer support groups, where they can both learn how others deal with a changed identity, compare their own situation, and continue to feel they can make a contribution. Some cancer support groups focus on simply providing a regular meeting where people with cancer can share experiences. Often professionals linked to a cancer centre or a palliative care service will facilitate these. Elsewhere the emphasis may be on self-help, through a well-developed voluntary organization that provides a range of services from information to advocacy, even training for patients to enable them to advocate for themselves if they wish. Here the focus is on empowering patients who have felt overwhelmed by their disease and are seeking to regain some control. The organization Cancerlink provides a directory of voluntary self-help and support groups. Active self-help groups can sometimes be perceived as challenging by professionals. The questioning they can promote can feel like criticism of a service that is struggling to cope with limited resources. Here there is a real need to be clear about the possibility of anger about the disease being projected onto the cancer service. A regular meeting between service providers and the voluntary organization, which provides a channel to deal with issues as they come up, can be helpful. Meetings set up only at times of crisis have to operate in a heated atmosphere, which makes dispassionate discussion very difficult.

A day-care service is another way of providing a new social group where members have in common the experience of advancing illness, however different their other social circumstances. Two observational studies of day care both comment on the way day care provided an 'alternative reality' (Lawton 2000) or a new 'normality' (Richardson 2001) for those attending. Lawton's participants seldom discussed the future, for it is this loss of future that particularly sets them apart from friends and acquaintances in their past. For Richardson's participants 'normality' seemed to consist of a structured opportunity to get out of the house, the potential for making new relationships and learning new skills, and a determination to divert from the illness that dominated life elsewhere. In day-care settings the deterioration of a fellow attendee can be challenging because of the reminder of the power of the illness. Staff in some settings may conceal or gloss over this despite the commitment to openness in palliative care philosophy. It can help if how such an event may be handled is discussed by the staff group when setting up the day-care service and monitored regularly to see whether the system devised meets the needs of attendees and staff.

While palliative day-care services expanded rapidly in the UK from 1980 to 2000 and were claimed to improve quality of life and increase time spent at home, models of care have been varied, not necessarily relating to an assessment of need and not rigorously evaluated. Higginson et al. (2000) are carrying out an evaluation of palliative day care and as part of this have examined what day-care services in a sample area of the UK are offering. They have found no clear distinction between medical and social approaches to care but different layers of activity provided in varying ways. Physical, social, and emotional support were a common base layer but then different services might offer a selection, including medical support, symptom control, creative activities, or therapy services. In the week the researchers surveyed the services, 25 per cent of patients had attended for over a year. This does raise the question of the objectives of the service and of the continued monitoring of need. Richardson (2001) pointed out from her study how difficult discharge might be for patients having become attached to a new social group.

Family culture and roles

In Western countries, thanks to improved living conditions and improved healthcare, most deaths now occur in old age, when people are less engaged in formal public roles, and even, because of declining functions, in private and familial roles. So their deaths may make less impact than a younger person's on their community and family. But we cannot necessarily assume this, because what is important is the actual role that person plays in the family and what the meaning for individuals in the family is of the advancing death.

> Ann Jones, aged 81, was now clearly very frail but still insisted that the family gather at her house once a month for Sunday lunch, though her daughters and daughters-in-law now prepared the meal. Her older, unmarried daughter, Jeanette, valued this tradition, still lived at home, and desperately wanted to maintain things 'as they always had been' for as long as possible. Her middle son, Paul, had always felt undervalued but paralysed by his imperious mother and the rest of the family and his wife longed for her mother-in-law's death, hoping at last for freedom from his damaging family.

Using a systems perspective we recognize that a change in one part of the system will reverberate through the whole system to different degrees. So some assessment of how roles are distributed in the family of the person with advanced cancer will help us in working appropriately with the social and emotional pain that changing roles may bring. Is the person with advanced cancer the one that acts as the link between family members? Mothers or oldest daughters often play this role in the majority white culture in the UK, as in Ann Jones' family. Are they the conciliator or the one who breaks tension by making people laugh? Vess *et al.* (1983–4), considering bereaved families, distinguished between person-oriented and position-oriented families, and their analysis has relevance for families before the death. They suggest that position-oriented families, where roles are ascribed on the basis of age and gender, rather than interest or ability, will adapt less well to crisis and new demands. Person-oriented families, where communication is open and roles are negotiated on the basis of achievement and not on culturally prescribed norms, are likely to deal more easily with the declining health of one member of the family system. It would be wrong to imply that there may not be considerable emotional pain in person-oriented families despite their adaptability. However there may be less social pain than in a position-oriented family, where resentment at the changes and at inability to sustain valued ways of operating may make the family feel they are failing to maintain what they see as a social norm.

Carers

Carers too have a changed identity. They may be struggling to sustain other commitments to a job or to other needy family members, or life may be 'on hold' as they put the needs of the dying person first. They may feel ambivalent about calling on professional help (Hull 1990).

> Mary was a lively, active woman in her sixties but small and overweight. She had cared lovingly for her husband who had lost the use of his legs but he was now too heavy for her to manage. She agreed to have two paid carers each evening to put him to bed and felt relieved that there would no longer be an undignified and exhausting struggle in the evening. On the first evening they came she showed them into the bedroom and then retreated to the kitchen and wept bitterly. She perceived that their coming marked a point at which the privacy of her home would be increasingly invaded and hammered home her husband's continuing deterioration.

Since the passing of the Carers (Recognition and Services) Act in 1995, carers in the UK who are providing 'regular and substantial care' have been entitled to a formal assessment of their ability to care and any support needed. But as Smith (2001) found in her research, it is the more long-standing carers who embrace the title of 'carer' and who grasp what is expected of them by professionals in terms of responsibility in that role. Newer carers might be much less clear and more diffident about asking for support for themselves as well as the ill person. Those who do make demands for themselves can be challenging to professionals.

> Jane and Richard had been married for two years when he developed cancer of the pancreas aged 27. They were young professionals and ambitious. Both were paragliding enthusiasts. As he became more ill and dependent he became quieter and more contemplative. After a few weeks of full-time caring, Jane announced that she wanted to go back to work. Richard's mother was available to look after him and in a short time he returned to his family home with Jane's agreement, to be cared for there by his mother until he died. Jane's behaviour was very difficult for many of the married women professionals involved in the care and for some of her friends and family. While they did not necessarily expect Jane to be a full-time carer, to be so ready, so cheerfully, to relinquish her 'wifely duty' totally did not accord with their expectations of a woman's roles. There was quite an expectation that she would pay the price by having a painful and guilty bereavement but Jane lived quite comfortably with her decision.

Sexuality

One area where the social impact of advanced cancer is still undervalued by professionals is the changes it brings in the life of the sick person and their sexual partner. The effect of surgery and drugs on sexual function is well established. For example, Stanford et al. (2000) showed that 24 months after surgery for prostate cancer, maintaining an erection was still a moderate to big problem for 42% of the men involved. What is also well established is that patients expect that professionals will bring this topic up if appropriate and professionals expect that patients will bring this topic up if they have a problem. So the issue frequently falls into the gap. A barrier for professionals is of course the sensitivity of this issue, a wish not to be intrusive or to seem to be making assumptions about this person's sexual life. Here there may be a value in breaking one of the standard rules of counselling—only ask one question at a time. Monroe (1993) suggests that a question like 'Has your illness changed your family relationships, your life as a couple, your ability to get close to each other physically?' signals that you are open to discussion about these issues. Then the dying person or their partner can choose to focus on the general family relationships aspect of the question or can use it as an opportunity to discuss any difficulties, whether practical or emotional.

> Mabel, aged 59, had bone metastases from her breast cancer. She and her husband were anxious about putting undue strain on her fragile bones but wanted to continue their active sexual life. They were able to do so after simple advice about appropriate positions.

Helpful resources in this area of care are the local psychosexual clinic or SPOD, the London–based, national Association to Aid the Sexual and Personal Relationships of

People with a Disability. This organization produces a number of leaflets and has a helpline for anyone, professionals and carers included, seeking advice.

Dependants

One of the most painful issues that those with advanced metastatic cancer may have to confront is the change the illness and their death will bring to those dependent upon them. The emotional distress for healthy, independent adults who love them may be hard enough to contemplate, how much more difficult to consider the losses for a vulnerable dependant. That person may be a child, or an adult with learning disabilities, or a frail, confused partner for whom the dying person has been the main carer. In all these situations there is a need for some preparation before the death and this of course may be particularly painful for a dying person who has been wishing to deny this possibility or at the least avoid discussing it. If after the death there will still be someone living in the same house who will continue to be able to care for the vulnerable person, for example the other parent, then it may be possible to offer the dying person some protection. What is then most important is that the vulnerable person is prepared for the change by the person who will continue the care. Where this element of continuity is not possible, preparation and planning for the transition are vital. All too often people with learning disabilities, for example, have been moved quite suddenly into a residential setting following the expected death of their carer with no recognition of their distress (Oswin 1991). The existence now of a National Network for the Palliative Care of People with Learning Disabilities and the growing number of research and practice projects in this field demonstrate that this group's needs are at last beginning to be addressed. It is important not to make assumptions about what they do or do not understand. Overprotection can be counterproductive. This was nicely demonstrated by a contributor to the national meeting of the network in November 2001 who had cared for her sister with learning disabilities. 'When our mother died I told her the angels had come to take her away. She was crying uncontrollably and when I asked her why she said "I want Mummy to have a proper coffin like everyone else".' Certainly children from the Liverpool Bereavement Project who drew up a leaflet for other bereaved children were clear. 'It's best to be involved in and given choices about how you say good bye' (Barnard *et al.* 1999).

There are a number of principles that are helpful to guide practice in supporting children facing the death of a parent, some of which apply equally well to other vulnerable groups.

1. **Find out what the child knows or believes about the situation.** Children pick up much more than adults think from overheard conversations, from atmospheres, and from what their friends have heard from their parents. They may not always interpret what they hear or perceive accurately—all the more reason for checking out that they are not inappropriately distressed, perhaps blaming themselves for causing the illness.

2. **Help parents to talk to their children.** They know their child best, and can take advantage of a good moment for a conversation. Sometimes they may need reassurance that this is good parenting, trying to give the child knowledge and a greater

sense of control in an uncontrollable situation. Sometimes they are keen to talk but uncertain how to go about it. So checking out with them what they think the child knows, offering support as they work out how to open up a discussion, and hearing how that went, are all valuable roles professionals can play. Clearly pacing and age-appropriate language must be considered. It is not necessary to tell children their mother is dying when her bone metastases have only just been picked up and it is likely that she will live for some time yet. It is important that they know that Mum and Dad are upset and distracted because the doctors have found some more signs of a serious illness.

3. **Help parents to consider what resources there might be within their family or community that could also be helpful to their children while they themselves have so much to cope with.** Schools can be very supportive but may also welcome some advice from palliative care professionals if they have not encountered this situation before. One important ethical principle here—consult children before talking to the school. Otherwise it may be more difficult if they are suddenly faced with the fact that their personal private grief is known by all.

4. **Use play.** There are many storybooks and workbooks now for children that can help them both to develop their understanding and express their feelings through art or games. *Finding a way through when someone close has died* (Mood and Whittaker 2001), produced by a group of young people, focuses most on the period after a death but has a list of books and resources, many of which are also useful beforehand.

Who has parental responsibility?

In the twenty-first century families are becoming ever more complex in their relationships. A couple may have come together, each bringing children from a previous relationship and then had children of their own. Marriage is becoming less common and it is now more usual for children to be born out of wedlock than in it. None of this may cause any problem unless the couple decides to separate or the partnership is threatened by advancing serious illness. Then who has parental responsibility and who does not may well become an issue. At the time of writing, the effective act is the Children Act (1989), though the Human Rights Act may in the end affect this. The Children Act (1989) changed rights to responsibilities. The mother always has parental responsibility. The father only has it if he was married to the mother when the child is born. He does not automatically acquire it even if he marries her subsequently. The non-married father can acquire parental responsibility in two ways. He and the mother can draw up a parental responsibility agreement made in the form prescribed by the Lord Chancellor and registered in the High Court or he can apply to the High Court to make a parental responsibility order in his favour. If the mother does not wish the father to have it, any other person with whom the child is living, for example grandparents, can apply for a residence order under the Children Act (1989) and through this acquire parental responsibility while the child continues to live with that person. Alternatively the mother can agree to a deed of guardianship before her death nominating whoever she feels suitable and can then bequeath her parental responsibility to that guardian. If a father is in dispute with a mother over this issue, he can take her to court and the court can make a parental responsibility or a residence order permitting the child to live with the father. With any family where parental responsibility is not straightforward these issues need to be considered, and for complex, reconstituted families early advice from a solicitor is vital.

> Yvonne and Peter had two children from their relationship, Paul, aged 5 and Vicky, aged 3. Yvonne also had a child by a previous relationship, Martin, aged 10, who saw his father intermittently and whose relationship with Peter was difficult. He often stayed with Yvonne's mother, who did not have a great deal of time for Peter. When it became clear Yvonne would die in the next few weeks from her cancer of the pancreas, Peter asked her to marry him. She refused. Her mother, an active 55-year-old, who had become increasingly distraught at the likely loss of her only child and fearful that she would lose all contact with her grandchildren once Yvonne died, was offering to look after all the children. Yvonne was worried that Peter would find another partner after her death who would not look after her children properly. In those circumstances she preferred her mother to care for them and talked of making a will in her favour. As she sank into a coma, battle raged between Peter and his family and Yvonne's mother and her family. The children's behaviour—Vicky wetting the bed again, Martin playing up at school, and Paul having nightmares—demonstrated the insecurity that they all felt. A much earlier discussion, which could have acknowledged some of the adults' fears and given time to work out a compromise, could have made this death much less horrific and divisive.

If parents are reluctant to tackle this issue because it feels like giving up the fight to acknowledge that one parent is dying, the strategy of 'what if' or 'hoping for the best and planning for the worst' can be helpful here. Confirming that while it may be important to continue to hope, and even struggle, for the best outcome, the professional can alongside this suggest that as good parents they may also want to prepare for the worst outcome so that the children are protected whatever the eventuality.

Who am I? What did I contribute?

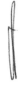

In an earlier section we looked at the challenges to identity that the losses of advancing cancer bring. For many these may be explored within a spiritual framework but there is also a social aspect to the challenge. This is a time when reviewing the past to put the present in context can be very affirming to the dying person. This may be done in several ways. For some people informal talk with family and friends may well give the opportunity to go over past triumphs and tragedies and to receive confirmation from them that their contribution has been valued. For others a more formal life review may be helpful in settling anxiety and uncertainty. Formal life review processes have been developed in many parts of the world following the seminal article by Butler (1963). Lichter (1993) trained volunteers in a New Zealand hospice to assist patients to complete oral or written accounts of their lives. Lester (1997) has built on the work of Haight *et al.* (1995) with older people in the USA to develop a structured questionnaire covering childhood, adult life, and the present for work with people with advancing illness. An improvement in life satisfaction and reduction in stress have been found following such a review. Reminiscence sessions in day care, encouraging members to bring materials focusing round a historical period like the Second World War or round a common interest such as fashions through the participants' lifetimes, can also provide an affirmation of the importance of an experience with others who have shared it.

What am I leaving behind?

Associated with life review can be a wish to leave a legacy or be involved in planing for the future of loved ones. Many patients value participating in creative activities in day care because it enables them to produce a painting or poem that provides concrete evidence of a contribution. A parent with young children who is dying may wish to leave a letter, an audio- or videotape for the children to keep and refer to as they grow up. The child welfare organization Barnardo's have produced a framework both for a 'memory book' and a 'memory box' to help parents and those working with them on this. It is important when embarking on such a project for the professional to be aware of some of the pitfalls. The dying parent will not be able to control how the memorial is kept or what use is made of it. Nor will it be helpful for the children to be too prescriptive about the future. To say 'I hope you keep a strong Christian faith' or 'I know the family business will be safe in your hands' may create a burden of guilt for the child in the future. Material which concentrates on demonstrating the value of the child for that parent and reminders of times they shared is likely to be greatly treasured.

Making a will is another way of ensuring that your wishes continue to carry weight after your death. As with sorting out parental responsibility, tackling this may feel like giving up or bringing death uncomfortably close. So the strategy recommended in that situation may be helpful here—focusing on planning for the worst while hoping for the best, so that the issue can then be set on one side. Legal advice should be sought in all cases, to avoid additional unnecessary distress for the bereaved, because the laws of inheritance are complex. An interesting project funding the appointment and training of funeral advisers in two hospices reinforced how problematic it can be to plan for an unwelcome future. It was clear that people were often misinformed and unaware of their rights, but referrals came slowly, though they came from both dying and bereaved people. The project did generate considerable interest and mixed feelings among staff (Heatley 2001).

Support services

Most people spend 90 per cent of the last year of their life at home and indeed wish to die at home. Grande *et al.* (1998) have reviewed the factors that make death at home more likely. These are

- the existence of a fit and well-supported family carer, particularly a woman partner
- being a man
- being in a higher socio-economic group
- being younger rather than older
- good symptom control.

Hinton (1994) in his longtitudinal study found that provision of social work support and improved day care increased the percentage of home deaths.

Grande *et al.* (1998) conclude that the number of home deaths is more likely to be increased by improving access to the services available for those in lower socio-economic groups and by enabling men to take on the carer role. Interestingly they found the one study that showed women and older people more likely to die at home came from Italy, so the cultural and family context may in fact be more significant than age or gender. The supportive and palliative care guidance from the National Institute of Clinical Excellence is likely to recommend that a range of social support services should be available in the cancer network, many of which have already been alluded to in this chapter. These range from the availability of respite care and personal and domestic support at home, 24 hours a day, to laundry and meals services, adapted housing, and training for carers in moving and handling. Hopefully it will identify the importance of support to maintain adolescent and young cancer patients and carers in education and suggest that each in-patient setting should have at least one member of staff who has had training in working with children who have a parent with cancer.

For some people with advanced cancer there may come a point when they can no longer manage at home even with support and they are faced with the particular social pain of having to consider moving into a residential home or nursing home. This is a further challenge to identity and can bring a real sense of bereavement as someone gives up the home in which perhaps children were born and grew up, in which every corner carries memories. Different countries have different arrangements for financing institutional care and the current debates in the UK provide a good example of some of the practical and symbolic issues at stake. Over the last fifteen year of the twentieth century there was huge shift, never democratically decided, in the provision of long-stay beds from the National Health Service to the social care providers, the local authorities, and voluntary and private homes. Because healthcare is free at the point of access and social care is means-tested, a generation that expected to receive free services 'from the cradle to the grave' suddenly found they had to pay, even if they required substantial care. This raised issues about reciprocal obligation in families and of equity and justice. Parents might expect and hope for care from their adult children as they become more disabled and wish to pass on a financial legacy to those they love; children may expect to receive some financial benefit from their parents' estate. Should family members be expected to support each other practically, emotionally, and financially? Is it just that a successful businessman should receive the profits from the sale of his mother's house and expect that the tax payers, some of whom may be much poorer than him, should cover the cost of her nursing home fees? Professionals working with someone with advanced cancer who is facing giving up their home may well find themselves caught up in these debates and in the anger and disagreement which they bring. These are intensified by the different approaches now being taken by the four countries within the UK.

Conclusion

A holistic approach to the care of people with advanced metastatic cancer must take into account the issues raised in this chapter to provide comprehensive care. Each team needs access to a specialist in these areas, who is most likely to be a social worker.

However each team member has to have some appreciation of the power of social pain and what may help to reduce its impact. Working in this area requires good negotiation skills, a breadth of understanding, stamina, and sensitivity but the benefits for patients and those close to them of providing good social care are high.

References

Barnard P, Morland I, Nagy J (1999). *Children, bereavement and trauma: nurturing resilience.* London: Jessica Kingsley.

Butler RN (1963). The life review: an interpretation of reminiscence in the aged. *Psychiatry* 26:65–73.

Donnelly S (1999). Folklore associated with dying in the west of Ireland. *Palliative Med* 13:57–62.

Field D (2000). What do we mean by 'psychosocial'? London: National Council for Hospice and Specialist Palliative Care Services. Briefing Paper No.4.

Firth S (1997). *Death, dying and bereavement in a British Hindu community.* Leuven: Peeters.

Firth S (2001). *Wider horizons: care of the dying in a multicultural society.* London: National Council for Hospice and Specialist Palliative Care Services.

Grande G, Addington-Hall J, Todd C (1998). Place of death and access to home care: are certain patient groups at a disadvantage? *Social Science Med* 47:565–79.

Haight B, Coleman P, Lord K (1995). The linchpins of successful life review: structure, evaluation and individuality. In: Haight B, Webster J (ed.). *The art and science of reminiscing: theory, research, methods and application.* Washington DC: Taylor and Francis, pp. 179–92.

Heatley R (2001). *Funeral advisors: is there a need? A pilot study.* Bristol: National Funerals College.

Higginson I, Hearn J, Myers K, Naysmith A (2000). Palliative day care: what do services do? *Palliative Med* 14:277–86.

Hinton J (1994). Which patients with terminal cancer are admitted from home care? *Palliative Med* 8:183–96.

Hull M (1990). Sources of stress for hospice-based care-giving families. In: Kirschling JM (ed.). *Family-based palliative care.* New York: Howarth, pp. 29–54.

Lawton J (2000). *The dying process: patients' experiences of palliative care.* London: Routledge.

Lester J (1997). Life review with the terminally ill. Proceedings of the Fourth Congress of the European Association for Palliative Care; 6–9 December 1995; Barcelona. Milan: European Association for Palliative Care.

Lichter I (1993). Biography as therapy. *Palliative Med* 7:133–7.

Mood P, Whittaker L (2001). *Finding a way through when someone close has died. A workbook by young people for young people.* London: Jessica Kingsley.

Monroe B (1993). Psychosocial dimension of palliation. In: Saunders C, Sykes N (ed.). *The management of terminal malignant disease.* London: Edward Arnold, pp. 174–201.

Myers K (2002). *Flying home—or on holiday.* Hospice Information: London. http://www.hospiceinformation.info.

National Institute of Clinical Excellence (in preparation). *Supportive and palliative care guidance: the manual.*

Neale B (1991). Informal palliative care. a review of research on needs, standards and service evaluation. Sheffield: Trent Palliative Care Centre. Occasional Paper No. 3.

Neuberger J (1993). Cultural issues in palliative care. In: Doyle D, Hanks G, Macdonald N. (ed.). *Oxford textbook of palliative medicine*. Oxford: Oxford University Press, pp. 507–513.

Oswin M (1991). *Am I allowed to cry? A study of bereavement among people who have learning difficulties*. London: Souvenir Press.

Richardson H (2001). A study of palliative day care using multiple case studies [presentation]. Palliative Care Research Forum, Royal College of Physicians; 7 June 2001; London.

Seale C, Addington-Hall J (1994). Euthanasia; why people want to die earlier. *Soc Sci Med* 39:647–54.

Smith P (2001). Who is a carer? Experiences of family caregivers in palliative care. In: Payne S, Ellis-Hill C (ed.). *Chronic and terminal illness: new perspectives on caring and carers*. Oxford: Oxford University Press, pp. 83–99.

Stanford J, Feng Z, Hamilton AS, Gilliland FD, Stephenson RA, Eley JW (2000). Urinary and sexual function after radical prostatectomy for clinically localised cancer. The prostate cancer outcomes study. *J Am Med Assoc* 283:354–60.

Stevenson O (1973). *Claimant or client?* London: Allen and Unwin.

Stroebe M (1998). New directions in bereavement research: exploration of gender differences. *Palliative Med* 12:5–12.

Sykes N, Pearson S, Chell S (1992). Quality of care: the carer's perspective. *Palliative Med* 6:227–36.

Vess J, Morland J, Schwebel A (1983–4). Understanding family role reallocation following a death. *Omega* 16:115–28.

Walter T (1994) *The revival of death*. London: Routledge.

Chapter 4

Current provision of psychosocial care within palliative care

Leslie Walker, Mary Walker, and
Donald Sharp

Introduction

Despite major advances in the treatment of many cancers and improvements in the delivery of palliative care, the diagnosis and treatment of cancer continue to cause wide-ranging types of distress and disruption to the lives of patients and their families. It is now universally accepted that many patients with cancer will experience a clinically significant psychological or psychiatric disorder at some point during their illness. In addition to impoverishing quality of life, treatment outcome and, ultimately, prognosis may be compromised by clinically significant psychological distress (Anderson and Walker 2002; Walker *et al.* 1999*a*).

Although the importance of information and support in alleviating distress is now accepted and the value of psychosocial interventions well documented in the literature, there is little agreement as to how psychosocial support services should be organized within a healthcare system such as the National Health Service (NHS). Should resources be used to prevent clinically significant distress and improve quality of life in the many or should they be concentrated on treating significant distress in the few? What is the place of group, as opposed to individual, interventions? How can staff be helped to provide support?

For the purposes of this chapter, psychosocial care will be defined as (National Council for Hospice and Specialist Palliative Care Services 1997)

> psychological approaches concerned with enabling patients and those close to them to express thoughts, feelings and concerns relating to illness, assessing their individual needs and resources and ensuring that psychological and emotional support is available. A range of informal and planned interventions may be used to relieve psychological distress, e.g. anxiety, anger, low mood and intrusive thoughts. For some patients this will also include the recognition and treatment of specific psychiatric disorders such as depressive illness.

This chapter aims to review the nature and prevalence of cancer-related distress, the evidence base for different types and levels of psychosocial interventions, and various options for delivering psychosocial support.

The nature and prevalence of psychological distress

A classic, US study (Derogatis *et al.* 1983) investigated the prevalence of psychiatric disorders in 215 randomly selected adult cancer patients with varying types and stages of disease. As many as 47 per cent of these patients were suffering from a diagnosable psychiatric disorder according to standardized criteria. Approximately 68 per cent of the psychiatric diagnoses consisted of adjustment disorders, with 13 per cent representing major affective disorders (depression). It is important to note that almost 90 per cent of the disorders did not predate the diagnosis of cancer, indicating that they were reactions to, or manifestations of, cancer or treatment.

In an earlier study in the UK, Maguire *et al.* (1978) found that in the year following surgery for breast cancer, 25 per cent of the women suffered from clinically significant anxiety or depression, and 33 per cent had moderate or severe sexual problems. The same group also found that as many as 81 per cent of a small series of women receiving adjuvant combination chemotherapy (Cyclophosphamide Methotrexate 5-Fluorouracil, CMF) for breast cancer developed a psychiatric disorder during treatment (Maguire *et al.* 1980a).

Recently, Zabora *et al.* (2001) assessed 4496 patients with differing types and stages of disease. Overall, 35 per cent of the sample were suffering from clinically significant levels of distress, which varied according to cancer type. The level of distress for patients with lung cancer was significantly higher than that for other cancers, with the exceptions of cancer of the brain, liver, pancreas, and head and neck. This recent study is important because the rates of distress were similar to those of the earlier studies discussed above.

The determinants of psychological distress

Harrison and Maguire (1994) reviewed predictors of psychological and psychiatric disorders in patients with cancer. They concluded that the following are risk factors: a previous history of mood disturbance, high emotionality, low ego strength, poor performance status ('fitness'), certain types of treatments (for example, colostomy), lack of social support, passive or avoidant coping, inadequate or inappropriate information, and communication problems. To this we might add the number of unresolved concerns (Worden and Weisman 1984) and the partner's distress level (Anderson *et al.* 2000).

Regarding treatment-related distress, it is well known that chemotherapy-related side-effects such as nausea, vomiting, alopecia, and fatigue are a common cause of distress (Bliss *et al.* 1992; Knobf *et al.* 1998). Considerable morbidity can also be caused by treatments such as radiotherapy (Chaturvedi *et al.* 1996; Greenberg 1998), surgery (Jacobsen and Hann 1998), bone marrow transplantion (Chiodi *et al.* 2000), and the biological response modifiers (Walker *et al.* 1996; Walker *et al.* 1997).

Several predictors of distress, such as a history of mood disturbance and performance status, cannot be altered. However, at least potentially, a number of these risk factors can be altered, for example, ego strength, coping style, extent of the partner's distress, amount of support, number of unresolved concerns, adequacy of information, and satisfaction with communication.

Information and support

In a study of 2027 patients with cancer in the UK, Jenkins *et al.* (2001) found that 98 per cent indicated that they preferred to know whether or not their diagnosis was cancer and 87 per cent said that they wanted all possible information, good or bad. Men were less likely than women to wish to know about all the possible treatments and older patients (over 70 years of age) were more likely to say that they preferred to leave disclosure of details to the doctors.

A number of studies have assessed the importance of information in helping patients to cope with the diagnosis and treatment of cancer (Walker 1996). For example, a follow-up study of 117 women attending a gynaecological oncology follow-up clinic indicated that those who were clinically anxious or depressed at follow-up were more critical of doctor–patient interaction, particularly regarding the amount of information given (Paraskevaidis *et al.* 1993). It should be borne in mind, however, that this study identified a small group of patients who felt that they would have coped better by having been told less and 13 per cent of the very large cohort studied by Jenkins *et al.* (2001 op. cit.) did *not* wish to be given all possible information.

It is clear that individuals differ in terms of what they wish to know, when they wish to be told, and from whom they wish to receive the information.

Historically, many patients have felt underinformed. Undoubtedly, information leaflets have become much more widely available in recent years. However, there is evidence that some patients find these of limited value and most prefer to receive information from healthcare professionals who can discuss the implications and answer questions (Farrell 2001). Also, services such as CancerBACUP have met and continue to meet otherwise unmet information needs. In the year 1999–2000, CancerBACUP distributed over 200 000 booklets and their website was visited by over 35 000 people per month.

Slevin *et al.* (1996) define emotional support as 'spending time with another person, listening and talking about problems and concerns in a way that is helpful and reassuring'. Recent studies in the UK have demonstrated that, currently, patients perceive lack of support to be a bigger problem than lack of information. For example, in a survey carried out in the East Riding of Yorkshire, UK in 1998, 120 patients with cancer were asked to look back on their treatment and identify one thing that they would wish to change (Thorpe 1998). Eighty-five per cent indicated that they wished to change some aspect of the care they had received. Twenty-eight per cent wanted improved support, whereas only 12 per cent wished for better information.

In a cross-sectional survey, Slevin *et al.* (1996) obtained the views of 431 patients about different sources of support and their satisfaction with these providers. They found that the three most important sources of support were senior registrars (73 per cent), family (73 per cent), and consultant staff (63 per cent). Forty-three per cent said they would definitely use their general practitioner (GP) as a source of support and, of those that had used their GP, 63 per cent were satisfied with the support received. Approximately eighty per cent were satisfied with the support received from senior medical staff, whereas only 42 per cent were satisfied with the support given by the ward nurses.

A study of 49 patients with orofacial cancers showed wide variation in the extent to which patients perceived primary and secondary care teams to be helpful (Broomfield *et al.* 1997). In keeping with the findings of Slevin *et al.* (1996), GPs were seen to be less helpful than family or hospital staff. Whereas 96 per cent found the support received by consultants to be helpful, only 50 per cent reported that they found support from the GP to be helpful; 10 per cent actually said the GPs support had been 'unhelpful' and four per cent indicated that it had been 'very unhelpful'.

Case study 1

With these considerations in mind, 12 years ago in Aberdeen a service was designed to minimize distress and improve quality of life. The result was a Behavioural Oncology Unit, which included a 'drop-in' centre that was fully integrated functionally, and physically, with the medical and surgical oncology services (Walker *et al.* 1999*a,b*).

A professional but informal atmosphere was cultivated—the kettle was always on. Patients and their relatives were welcome to visit or telephone at any time. We gave our staff special training to make sure that they had the skills necessary to elicit cancer-related concerns and, equally importantly, to respond effectively to these (Maguire *et al.* 1996). We customized the information given. We provided the opportunity for peer-group and staff support and, as far as patients were concerned, psychosocial support and medical and surgical treatments were seamlessly integrated. The unit was located within the Professorial Surgical Unit and patients received their chemotherapy under the supervision of a consultant medical oncologist within the Behavioural Oncology Unit. It was possible for us to make sure that, from the patient's point of view, investigations and treatments were carried out with the minimum delay; the minimum fuss, and the maximum coordination.

A consecutive series of 96 women attending the unit because of newly diagnosed locally advanced breast cancer were studied intensively over a period of 37 weeks (Walker *et al.* 1999*a*). They were assessed using a number of tests, including the hospital anxiety and depression scale (HADS) (Zigmond and Snaith 1983). Immediately after the diagnosis had been made, when they were in-patients in the Professorial Surgical Unit, waiting to start their chemotherapy, 21 per cent scored 11 or above on the anxiety sub-scale of the HADS. This is usually taken to indicate clinically significant anxiety. However, surveys of other groups of women in the north-east of Scotland, for example, surveys of police officers, psychiatric nurses, and wives of police officers, had consistently found a point prevalence of 15–25 per cent (see, for example, Alexander *et al.* 1993). These women with newly diagnosed breast cancer were undoubtedly 'stressed', but they were not clinically 'distressed'.

Eighteen weeks later, having had six cycles of chemotherapy and whilst awaiting surgery, the point prevalence had fallen to five per cent. This is obviously much lower than it had been at diagnosis, and much lower than it was in the so-called healthy population of the north-east of Scotland.

Thirty-seven weeks after the diagnosis, following chemotherapy, surgery, hormone therapy, and radiotherapy, the point prevalence had fallen further to a very striking two per cent and other psychometric tests, and structured clinical interviews using standardized psychiatric criteria, confirmed the low rate of morbidity.

These data suggest that by providing a functionally and topographically integrated psychosocial support service, patients can be mentally healthier than they were before treatment and mentally healthier than 'healthy' women in the community.

Randomized, controlled trials of psychosocial interventions

Five meta-analyses (of variable quality) have been published (Devine and Westlake 1995; Luebbert et al. 2001; Meyer and Mark 1995; Smith et al. 1994; Sheard and Maguire 1999), which suggest that a range of psychosocial interventions have beneficial effects on emotional adjustment, function, treatment-related side-effects (especially nausea and vomiting), pain, and global quality of life.

Interventions to reduce distress and improve adaptation in unselected patients

It has been argued that healthcare professionals should direct their attention to only those patients who are showing clinically significant levels of distress and it has also been suggested that randomized trials to evaluate psychological interventions should concentrate on such individuals, not least because effects will be easier to demonstrate (see, for example, Baider et al. 2001; Sheard and Maguire 1999). However, the following randomized trials show that benefits to unselected groups of patients with cancer can be demonstrated.

Maguire et al. (1980b) randomized 152 women with breast cancer either to specialist counselling from a breast care nurse or to routine practice. Counselling by a specialist nurse did not prevent psychiatric morbidity, although this regular monitoring resulted in the referral of 76 per cent of those who needed psychiatric help to an appropriate agency. Only 15 per cent of the control group whose condition merited referral were recognized and referred. Consequently, at follow-up, the patients who had been randomized to the specialist nurse were less likely to suffer from a psychiatric disorder than those who received standard care (12 per cent compared with 39 per cent). Subsequently, Maguire et al. (1983) showed that patients randomized to the specialist nurse had improved marital and sexual adjustment, they were more likely to return to work, and they were more satisfied with their prosthesis. However, there was only a limited effect on physical symptoms.

In another evaluation study of specialist nurses, Watson et al. (1988) randomized 40 newly diagnosed breast cancer patients who had undergone mastectomy to routine care or to routine care plus counselling by a nurse. Although there were some initial advantages for those receiving counselling, there were no significant differences between the two groups 12 months post-operatively. The authors interpret these findings as suggesting that a nurse counselling service can speed up the process of adjustment following surgery.

A more recent study (McArdle *et al.* 1996) compared support from a breast care nurse specialist with voluntary support. Two-hundred-and-seventy-two patients were randomized to routine care from ward staff, routine care plus support from the breast care nurse, routine care plus support from a voluntary organization, or routine care plus support from the nurse and the voluntary organization. Measures of anxiety and depression were consistently lower in patients who were offered support from the breast care nurse. The authors concluded that support from this breast care nurse significantly reduced psychological morbidity, as measured by self-rating scales. The study, however, has been criticized for various reasons, including the fact that only one breast care nurse was used in the study and the voluntary organization was restricted in terms of the interventions it was able to offer.

In the USA, a number of authors have argued that group, as opposed to, individual, interventions are particularly beneficial. Spiegel *et al.* (1981) randomized 86 women with metastatic breast cancer to group support or standard care. The groups focused on the problems of terminal illness and associated interpersonal consequences, as well as living as fully as possible in the face of death. Hypnosis and relaxation were also used as appropriate. The data showed that patients receiving group support had fewer maladaptive coping responses and less mood disturbance than those in the standard care arm of the trial.

The effects of a different type of group intervention were evaluated by Fawzy *et al.* (1990). They randomized 68 patients with newly diagnosed malignant melanoma to a brief (once weekly for six weeks) psycho-educational intervention consisting of health education, enhancement of problem-solving skills, stress management (including relaxation techniques), and support. When the patients were followed up six months later, patients randomized to the intervention showed significantly less depressed mood, fatigue, confusion, and total mood disturbance. They also used more active–behavioural and active–cognitive coping methods than the control participants.

The *Starting again programme* developed by Berglund *et al.* (1994) also has a strong educational component. Two-hundred-and-ninety-two patients with various cancer diagnoses who had completed post-operative adjunctive treatment within the previous two months were invited to participate. One-hundred-and-ninety-nine agreed to be randomized. The programme involved 11 two-hour sessions over a period of seven weeks and consisted of physical training, education (cancer, treatments, and diets), and practical problem solving (including coping with the reactions of other people, anxiety, and medical reviews). Compared with control participants, patients in the *Starting again programme* showed better physical function, sleep, and body image. They also showed greater fighting spirit and were more satisfied with information.

Relaxation therapy is widely used in the UK and a number of randomized trials have been reported. Walker *et al.* (1999a) examined the effects of relaxation therapy with guided imagery (visualizing host defences attacking cancer cells or in some other way promoting 'healing') in 96 women receiving combination neoadjuvant (primary) chemotherapy for newly diagnosed locally advanced breast cancer. They found that relaxation and guided imagery were acceptable to most patients. When the data were analysed using a conservative intention-to-treat method, patients randomized to relaxation and guided imagery reported significantly better quality of life during chemotherapy and they were more relaxed and more easy going as assessed using the mood rating scale. The intervention also reduced emotional suppression. Intriguingly, patient self-rated imagery vividness correlated significantly with clinical response to neoadjuvant chemotherapy. It is interesting to note that there was no significant difference in the incidence of clinically significant depression or anxiety, presumably for the reasons given in the case study above.

Cunningham *et al.* (1995) addressed the interesting issue of how best to schedule interventions. They compared a brief group psycho-educational programme delivered as six weekly two-hour sessions with a 'weekend intensive'. One-hundred-and-fifty-six patients were randomized. The weekend intensive produced a rapid, large improvement in mood, although the two interventions did not differ with respect to mood after six weeks and 19 weeks. At six weeks, patients in the six-week programme had better quality of life, although the difference between the interventions had disappeared by 19 weeks. The authors conclude that the two interventions are broadly comparable. They make the valuable point that there is a 'particular need for ways of bringing the benefits of psychosocial help to a larger population, including people of varying ethnic backgrounds. This will probably mean adapting both the format and the content of programs to suit consumer's needs, and integrating this adjunctive help more closely into the overall medical treatment scheme.' The issue of equity of use is a very important one which is addressed in detail later in this chapter.

Brief, 'low-key' interventions have also been shown to be beneficial in unselected patients. McQuellon (1998) randomly assigned 150 consecutively referred patients to an oncology out-patient clinic to usual care or to an intervention consisting of a clinic tour, information about the clinic, and a question-and-answer session. At follow-up, those randomized to the intervention programme had a lower state of anxiety, lower overall distress, and a reduced incidence of depressive symptoms. The patients were also more knowledgeable about clinic procedures and were more satisfied with the care they had received.

Another successful, 'low-key' intervention was evaluated by Burton *et al.* (1995) who examined the possible benefits of presurgical interventions. Two hundred women scheduled for mastectomy were randomized to one of four interventions: preoperative interview plus a 30 minute psychotherapeutic intervention, preoperative interview plus a 'chat' (to control for attention), preoperative interview only, and routine care. The preoperative interview covered the discovery of the breast problem, referral, beliefs about the causes of the illness, response to the need for surgery, desire for information, worries about body image, support, life events, and attitude to the past and the future. A brief structured psychiatric interview was also carried out. Patients receiving a preoperative interview showed less body image disturbance than the patients receiving standard care three months and 12 months after surgery. Compared with the three intervention groups, patients receiving routine care were more likely to have clinically significant anxiety and depression 12 months after surgery, and they also scored lower on 'fighting spirit'. Interestingly, psychological morbidity was 59 per cent preoperatively and 39 per cent one year after surgery. This study highlights the value of a preoperative interview in terms of long-term adjustment.

In addition to improving various aspects of coping and quality of life, psychosocial interventions can also modify various behaviours relevant to treatment outcome. For example, Richardson *et al.* (1990) reported a very interesting study on the effects of three special educational programmes and treatment compliance in 96 patients with haematological malignancies. The educational programmes involved helping the patients to develop a routine for taking medication, educating the patients regarding the importance of treatment compliance and self-care, and a behavioural-shaping programme. All three programmes increased treatment compliance (and survival), indicating that treatment compliance can be improved by means of relatively simple interventions.

These studies allow two general conclusions. First, relatively brief, simple interventions, delivered individually or in a group, can reduce distress and improve quality of life in patients who have not been selected because they have clinically significant distress, or who are at high risk of developing such distress. Second, although it may be more difficult to demonstrate between-group differences, it is possible to demonstrate these effects in unselected populations using the methodological gold standard, namely the prospective, randomized, controlled trial (Walker and Anderson, 1999).

In the next section, evidence for the benefits of psychosocial interventions in distressed populations is reviewed.

Interventions for patients with clinically significant problems

Many studies have shown clear benefits of psychological interventions in patients suffering from various types of treatment-related distress. These have been reviewed recently by Redd *et al.* (2001) who identified 54 studies (not all of which were randomized trials). They concluded that behavioural interventions can effectively control anticipatory nausea and vomiting in adult and paediatric cancer patients undergoing chemotherapy; that they can ameliorate anxiety and distress associated with invasive medical treatments, and that hypnotic-like methods (relaxation, suggestion, and distracting imagery) are helpful for pain management. Specific illustrative examples of randomized, clinical trials are reported below.

To study the effectiveness of preventive intervention in lowering emotional distress and improving coping, Worden and Weisman (1984) assessed 381 newly diagnosed cancer patients. Fifty-nine patients predicted by a screening instrument to be at risk for high levels of emotional distress and poor coping were randomly allocated to one of two interventions designed to enhance problem-solving skills. A non-randomized control group (58 patients) received no intervention. Both interventions reduced emotional distress and improved problem resolution. Although only partially randomized, this influential early study suggests the value of a brief intervention in preventing distress and enhancing coping in high-risk patients.

In a large, prospective, randomized, controlled trial, Greer *et al.* (1992) evaluated the effect on quality of life of a brief, problem-based, cognitive–behavioural treatment specifically designed for the needs of patients with cancer (adjunctive psychological therapy (APT)). One-hundred-and-seventy-four patients who scored above a predetermined cut-off on two measures of psychological morbidity were recruited from 1260 patients who had been screened. High-scoring patients were randomized to standard care or to APT.

At eight-week follow-up, compared with the control patients, patients receiving APT were significantly better than control patients on fighting spirit, helplessness, anxious preoccupation, fatalism, anxiety, psychological symptoms, and healthcare orientation. Some of these gains persisted: at four months, compared with control patients, patients receiving APT were significantly less anxious, had fewer psychological symptoms, and had less psychological distress. Clinically, the proportion of severely anxious patients dropped from 46 per cent at baseline to 20 per cent at eight weeks and 20 per cent at four months in the therapy group and from 48 per cent to 41 per cent and 43 per cent respectively in the control group. The proportion of patients with depression was 40 per cent at baseline, 13 per cent at eight weeks, and 18 per cent at four months in the therapy group and 30 per cent, 29 per cent, and 23 per cent respectively in the control group.

When the patients were followed up after 12 months, patients were less anxious and depressed (Moorey *et al.* 1994). This study shows that, in a mixed group of distressed cancer patients, a brief intervention can improve various key components of quality of life.

Current psychosocial provision

It might be rightly said that psychosocial care is the business of all healthcare professionals who are in contact with patients who have cancer, their carers, and their relatives. However, across the UK, very little is known about the number and professional backgrounds of healthcare staff that have a particular responsibility for the provision of psychosocial care for patients with cancer and their relatives, in hospital or in the community. In addition, little is known about the training they have had in the provision of psychosocial care, how standards are monitored, and the support that they, themselves, receive to prevent 'burn-out' (Ramirez *et al.* 1995; Wilkinson 1995).

Lloyd-Williams *et al.* (1999) carried out a survey of psychosocial provision within hospices in the UK. One-hundred-and-sixty hospices were selected and a questionnaire sent to the matron or nurse-in-charge. Ninety-seven (60 per cent) of the questionnaires were returned. The majority (83 per cent) of hospices employed a chaplain and all had access to a chaplain if required. Seventy-five per cent employed a social worker and all but six per cent had access to one. Forty-three per cent employed one or more 'counsellors', although 25 per cent indicated that they did not have access to a counsellor. The most interesting findings, however, are that only nine per cent employed a full- or part-time psychiatrist and only seven per cent employed a psychologist. The authors conclude that treatable psychiatric morbidity may go undetected and untreated as a result.

Certainly, outside hospices, increasing numbers of specialist nurses, at least part of whose remit is the provision of psychosocial care, are being employed in hospitals and in the community throughout the UK. For example, the first Macmillan nursing posts were established in 1975. Currently, there are over 2000 Macmillan nurses in posts in almost every local health authority in the UK. In addition, the medical services programme was set up in 1986 to establish Macmillan doctors at all levels and roles, in hospitals, at home, and in cancer treatment centres and, to date, over 300 Macmillan doctors have been appointed. Macmillan Cancer Relief's contribution to cancer care in the UK is now widely recognized by the public and the NHS.

A widely reported problem with information and support services in the UK is that these services are used disproportionately by middle-class women with breast cancer. For example, a survey of clients accessing CancerBACUP, the Macmillan Lynda Jackson Centre, and the Richard Dimbleby Centre found that only 23–29 per cent of those contacting these services were men (Williams *et al.* 2000).

Non-equity of use was also found by Boudioni *et al.* (2000). They reviewed the socio-demographic data from all 384 clients who had booked an appointment with the Cancer BACUP London Counselling Service during a period of 18 months. The clients were predominantly women, under 50 years of age, and from non-manual social classes.

The situation in Germany has been studied by Plass and Koch (2001). One-hundred-and-thirty-two patients attending four oncology out-patient clinics in Hamburg completed a questionnaire to establish their knowledge of institutions offering support, their previous participation in support, their reasons for participation, and their evaluation of the support given. Eighty-eight per cent of the respondents were women and 72 per cent had a history of breast cancer. Twenty-eight per cent of the respondents had participated in some sort of psychosocial support (only 4 per cent of these had attended self-help groups). Those who had participated were younger and scored higher on measures of emotional and physical difficulties. The main reason for non-participation was the presence of adequate support from family, friends, or doctors.

A recent US study surveyed a randomly selected group of patients with breast, colon, or prostate cancer (Eakin and Strycker 2001). Use of all support and information services (hospital, community, the Internet) was low (2–8 per cent). The most common reasons for not using the hospital counselling service was adequate support, lack of awareness of the service, and not having been referred. Better-educated patients were more likely to use the hospital counselling service. Awareness of the prostate support group was high (90 per cent), although use was low (5 per cent).

Earlier in this chapter, we reviewed some of the evidence demonstrating that individual and group interventions both have beneficial effects on quality of life. However, they may differ markedly in terms of acceptability. Baider *et al.* (2001) reported that 90 out of 116 (78 per cent) eligible patients in Jerusalem agreed to participate in their randomized trial of progressive muscular relaxation and guided imagery in groups. Cultural factors may affect acceptability and group interventions themselves may differ in acceptability, for example, group psycho-educational approaches versus group supportive–expressive methods. Further research is required to clarify these issues.

In conclusion, the challenge is how best to organize psychosocial care in order to provide appropriate information and support to all patients (and relatives); to deliver patient-centred care; to prevent psychological morbidity; to improve quality of life; to work in partnership; and to reduce health inequalities.

Case study 2

In an attempt to minimize distress and enhance quality of life following the diagnosis of cancer, an Oncology Health Centre was recently established in Kingston-upon-Hull, UK. The service is based on research that we had carried out in Aberdeen (see case study 1 above). The aims of the service are

(1) to prevent psychological problems and to enhance quality of life;

(2) to provide a high-quality, integrated, evidence-based, multi-disciplinary clinical service for in-patients and out-patients with any type of cancer, and their families;

(3) to provide the opportunity to learn self-help techniques, such as relaxation and guided imagery;

(4) to carry out research into psychosocial aspects of understanding and treating cancer;

(5) to work closely with others involved in psychosocial support and to offer them clinical supervision and other opportunities for professional development;

(6) to provide local and national training programmes (physicians, surgeons, psychiatrists, psychologists, nurses, and therapists).

All patients with cancer and their relatives can 'drop in' to the centre. The atmosphere is informal and welcoming. Patients can also obtain information and support by telephoning the centre. In addition, any healthcare professional can refer patients who are experiencing particular difficulties.

Currently, up to 250 patients and relatives attend the centre each week and the number continues to increase.

The service comprises a nurse-led 'drop-in centre', which offers open access to all patients with a cancer diagnosis and their relatives and a psychologist-led service to which any healthcare professional, in hospital or in the community, can refer patients or relatives for evidence-based interventions. A key feature is that the centre is fully integrated functionally and topographically with mainstream oncological provision.

Psychosocial support can be considered in terms of a pyramid, where basic support is available to all (the bottom of the pyramid) and interventions become increasingly sophisticated and focused on those that need them towards the top of the pyramid. The model as applied to the Oncology Health Centre is shown in Fig. 4.1.

Patient centredness

The Oncology Health Centre aims to promote a patient-centred approach by

(1) giving support, information and advice in the context of a multi-disciplinary team and in an informal, welcoming atmosphere;

(2) providing open access (by telephone or in person) to individually tailored information about disease, symptoms, and side-effects;

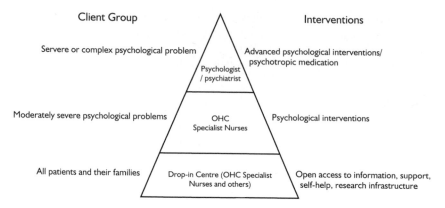

Fig. 4.1 Organisation of services within the Oncology Health Centre, Kingston-upon-Hull, UK.

(3) giving patients and relatives the opportunity to meet other patients and relatives;

(4) training staff to elicit and resolve concerns;

(5) offering evidence-based, self-help interventions, for example, relaxation and guided imagery.

Working in partnership

The centre is adjacent to the oncology and radiotherapy departments at the Princess Royal Hospital in Kingston-upon-Hull. This makes it very easy for centre staff to liaise with medical, radiological, and nursing staff. The location of the centre makes it convenient for patients to 'drop in' when they attend for radiotherapy, chemotherapy, or follow-up appointments. A key feature of the centre, therefore, is functional and topographical integration with other aspects of the oncology services. Oncologists, nurses, and radiotherapists often bring patients along to the centre personally. A leaflet describing what the centre offers is now given to most patients at the time of diagnosis and it is available at out-patient clinics and elsewhere.

The centre is staffed by two part-time consultant clinical psychologists, two part-time clinical psychologists, and four specialist behavioural oncology nurses (all funded by Hull and East Yorkshire Hospitals NHS Trust).

Tackling and reducing health inequalities

We have analysed the Townsend deprivation scores (Townsend *et al.* 1988) of the first 856 patients who attended the Oncology Health Centre and for whom Townsend deprivation scores were available from the 1991 census data. The scores are derived from postcodes. The Townsend ranks are as follows:

- ◆ rank 1 (most deprived)   34.4 per cent
- ◆ rank 2   23.3 per cent
- ◆ rank 3   12.0 per cent

- rank 4   13.8 per cent
- rank 5 (least deprived)   16.5 per cent.

These data show that 59 per cent of our patients came from the two most deprived groups (ranks 1 and 2), thereby demonstrating that the service is used widely by disadvantaged groups.

Analysis of the diagnoses of these 856 patients indicated that patients with all types of cancer attended.

Service evaluation

Nine months after the centre opened, a consecutive series of 51 patients and 38 relatives who had visited the centre at least once completed anonymously a satisfaction questionnaire. On average, they had visited the centre seven times (range 2–20). They were asked to indicate the extent to which they agreed or disagreed with various propositions. All agreed with the statements

- 'overall, I am satisfied with the care I have received in the Oncology Health Centre'
- 'I received a warm welcome'
- 'the staff understood my concerns'
- 'the staff responded helpfully to my concerns'
- 'I found it useful to talk to with the nurses in the centre'
- 'I feel the doctors and nurses in the Oncology Health Centre provide a valuable service'
- 'I consider the Oncology Health Centre provides a unique dimension of care'.
  Ninety-six per cent agreed with the statement
- 'I found it useful to talk with other patients'.

Challenging traditional boundaries

Patients are free to drop in to the centre, or to telephone, at any time during normal working hours. There is evidence that the number of unresolved concerns that patients have is a good predictor of subsequent distress (Heaven and Maguire 1998; Maguire *et al.* 1996). Frequently, patients are concerned about matters that can only be resolved by reference to the case notes or by contacting another member of the team. For this reason, topographical and functional integration is very important. The Oncology Health Centre is an attempt to put these principles into practice.

Working together

Several months after the centre opened, we sent a questionnaire to individuals who had referred one or more patients to the Oncology Health Centre. The 38 referrers who responded anonymously had referred 369 patients (a mean of 9.7 patients). The professional backgrounds of the referrers were as follows:

- hospital and community nurses   42 per cent
- physicians   28 per cent

- surgeons   17 per cent
- other medical staff   8 per cent
- social workers   3 per cent
- professions allied to medicine   3 per cent.

All believed the centre made a useful contribution to the overall care of patients with cancer and their relatives and were satisfied with the speed of the response to the referral and with the documentation they subsequently received. Ninety-seven per cent felt that what happened in the centre provided a unique dimension of care.

Soon after the service was established, a number of nurses asked for regular supervision and support from the two consultant clinical psychologists in the centre. A total of 33 specialist nurses from the local hospitals and from the community now receive regular supervision (in five groups).

Conclusions

The Oncology Health Centre at the Princess Royal Hospital, Kingston-upon-Hull is a novel, integrated approach to providing additional opportunities for psychosocial support. In future, we hope to set up a community network by establishing three small drop-in centres in the East Riding of Yorkshire and North Lincolnshire. These centres will be nurse led and will have video-conferencing links to the Oncology Health Centre. This will mean that patients and relatives will be able to obtain advice from specialist nurses and psychologists without having to travel to Kingston-upon-Hull.

Overall conclusions

It is clear that a great deal can be done to help patients with cancer and their relatives, ranging from the provision of appropriate information and support to the application of sophisticated psychosocial interventions. It is not clear to what extent these latter interventions are currently available in Europe and the USA and there is a need for a systematic survey of providers in order to ascertain who is providing what, and with what background, training, supervision, and support; we are currently planning such a survey in the UK.

Currently, services are organized in disparate ways and there is a pressing need to evaluate different models of service delivery in order to compare efficacy, effectiveness, and cost effectiveness. In addition, there is a need in the UK to coordinate, or network, the services provided by various individuals providing psychosocial support in hospitals and in the community.

Perhaps psychosocial support services should be considered analogously to items on a restaurant menu. Needs and desires differ. The challenge for psychosocial support services in the future is for them to be sufficiently well organized and networked so that all patients are aware of everything on the menu and sufficiently flexible to allow patients (and relatives) to choose what they need at any given time in their journey.

References

Alexander DA, Walker LG, Innes GW, Irving BL (1993). *Police stress at work.* London: Police Foundation.

Anderson J, Walker MB, Walker LG (2000). Distress and concerns of the partners of patients with breast cancer who receive primary chemotherapy. *Psycho-Oncology* **9**:357.

Anderson J, Walker LG (2002). Psychological factors and cancer progression: involvement of behavioural pathways. In: Lewis CE, O'Brien R, Barraclough J (ed.). *The psychoimmunology of Cancer.* 2nd edn. Oxford: Oxford University, pp. 235–57.

Baider L, Peretz T, Hadani PE, Koch U (2001). Psychological intervention in cancer patients: a randomized study. *Gen Hosp Psychiat* **23**:272–7.

Berglund G, Bolund C, Gustafsson U-L, Sjödén P-O (1994). A randomized study of a rehabilitation programme for cancer patients: the 'starting again' group. *Psycho-oncology* **3**:109–20.

Bliss JM, Robertson B, Selby PJ (1992). The impact of nausea and vomiting upon quality of life measures. *Br J Cancer* **66** (**suppl XIX**):S14–23.

Boudioni M, Mossman J, Boulton M, Ramirez A, Moynihan C, Leydon G (2000). An evaluation of a cancer counselling service. *Eur J Cancer* **9**:212–20.

Broomfield D, Humphris GM, Fisher SE, Vaughan D, Brown JS, Lane S (1997). The orofacial cancer patient's support from the general practitioner, hospital teams, family, and friends. *J Cancer Ed* **12**:229–32.

Burton MV, Parker RW, Farrell A, Bailey D, Connely J, Booth S *et al.* (1995). A randomized controlled trial of preoperative psychological preparation for mastectomy. *Psycho-oncology* **4**:1–19.

Chaturvedi SK, Chandra PS, Channabasavanna SM, Anantha N, Reddy BKM, Sharme S (1996). Levels of anxiety and depression in patients receiving radiotherapy in India. *Psycho-oncology* **5**:343–6.

Chiodi S, Spinelli S, Ravera G, Petti AR, Van Lint MT, Lamparelli T *et al.* (2000). Quality of life in 244 recipients of allogeneic bone marrow transplantation. *Br J Haematol* **110**:614–19.

Cunningham AJ, Jenkins G, Edmonds CV, Lockwood GA (1995). A randomised comparison of two forms of a brief, group, psychoeducational program for cancer patients: weekly sessions versus a 'weekend intensive'. *Int J Psychiat Med* **25**:173–89.

Derogatis LR, Morrow GR, Fetting JH, Penman D, Piatsky S, Schmale AM *et al.* (1983). The prevalence of psychiatric disorders amongst cancer patients. *J Am Med Assoc* **249**:751–7.

Devine EC, Westlake SK (1995). The effects of psychoeducational care provided to adults with cancer: meta-analysis of 116 studies. *Oncology Nursing Forum* **22**:1369–81.

Eakin EG, Strycker LA (2001). Awareness and barriers to use of cancer support and information resources by HMO patients with breast, prostate, or colon cancer: patient and provider perspectives. *Psycho-oncology* **10**:103–13.

Farrell C (2001). National service framework Assessments No. 1: NHS cancer care in England and Wales. London: Commission for Health Improvement. Supporting Paper 1: There's no system to the whole procedure.

Fawzy FI, Cousins N, Fawzy NW, Kemeny ME, Elashoff R, Morton D (1990). A structured psychiatric intervention for cancer patients. I. Changes over time in methods of coping and affective disturbance. *Arch Gen Psychiat* **47**:720–5.

Greenberg DB (1998). Radiotherapy. In: Holland JC (ed.). *Psycho-Oncology.* New York: Oxford University Press, pp. 269–76.

Greer S, Moorey S, Baruch JDR, Watson M, Robertson BM, Mason A *et al.* (1992). Adjuvant psychological therapy for patients with cancer: a prospective randomised trial. *BMJ* 304:675–80.

Harrison J, Maguire P (1994). Predictors of psychiatric morbidity in cancer patients. *Br J Psychiat* 165:593–8.

Heaven CM, Maguire P (1998). The relationship between patients' concerns and psychological distress in a hospice setting. *Psycho-Oncology* 7:502–7.

Jacobsen PB, Hann DM (1998). Cognitive–behavioural interventions. In: Holland JC (ed.). *Psycho-Oncology.* New York: Oxford University Press, pp. 717–29.

Jenkins V, Fallowfield L, Saul J (2001). Information needs of patients with cancer: results from a large study in UK cancer centre. *Br J Cancer* 84:48–51.

Knobf MT, Pasacreta JV, Valentine A, McCorkle R (1998). Chemotherapy, hormone therapy, and immunotherapy. In: Holland JC (ed.). *Psycho-Oncology.* New York: Oxford University Press, pp. 277–88.

Lloyd-Williams M, Friedman T, Rudd N (1999). A survey of psychosocial service provision within hospices. *Palliative Med* 3:431–2.

Luebbert K, Dahme B, Hasenbring M (2001). The effectiveness of relaxation training in reducing treatment-related symptoms and improving emotional adjustment in acute non-surgical cancer treatment: a meta-analytical review. *Psycho-Oncology* 10:490–502.

Maguire GP, Lee EG, Bevington DJ, Kuchemann CS, Crabtree RJ, Cornell CE (1978). Psychiatric problems in the first year after mastectomy. *BMJ* 1:963–5.

Maguire GP, Tait A, Brooke M, Thomas C, Howat JM, Sellwood RA *et al.* (1980) Psychiatric morbidity and physical toxicity associated with adjuvant chemotherapy after mastectomy. *BMJ* 281:1179–80.

Maguire P, Tait A, Brooke M, Thomas C, Sellwood R (1980). Effect of counselling on the psychiatric morbidity associated with mastectomy. *BMJ* 281:1454–7.

Maguire P, Brooke M, Tait A, Thomas C, Sellwood R (1983). The effect of counselling on physical disability and social recovery after mastectomy. *Clin Oncol* 9:319–24.

Maguire P, Faulkner A, Booth K, Elliott C, Hillier V (1996). Helping cancer patients disclose their concerns. *Eur J Cancer* 32A:78–81.

McArdle JMC, George WD, McArdle CS, Smith DC, Moodie AR, Hughson AVM *et al.* (1996). Psychological support for patients undergoing breast cancer surgery: a randomised study. *BMJ* 312:813–16.

McQuellon RP, Wells M, Hoffman S, Craven B, Russell G, Cruz J *et al.* (1998). Reducing distress in cancer patients with an orientation program. *Psycho-oncology* 7:207–17.

Meyer TJ, Mark MM (1995). Effects of psychosocial interventions with adult cancer patients: a meta-analysis of randomized experiments. *Health Psychol* 14:101–8.

Moorey S, Greer S, Watson M, Baruch JDR, Robertson BM, Mason A *et al.* (1994). Adjuvant psychological therapy for patients with cancer: outcome at one year. *Psycho-oncology* 3:39–46.

National Council for Hospice and Specialist Palliative Care (1997). Feeling better: Psychosocial care in specialist palliative care. London: Occasional paper no. 13.

Paraskevaidis E, Kitchener HC, Walker L G (1993). Doctor–patient communication and subsequent mental health in women with gynaecological cancer. *Psycho-oncology* 2:195–200.

Plass A, Koch U (2001). Participation of oncological outpatients in psychosocial support. *Psycho-Oncology* 10:511–20.

Ramirez AJ, Graham J, Richards MA, Cull A, Gregory WM, Leaning MS *et al* (1995). Burnout and psychiatric disorder among cancer clinicians. *Br J Cancer* **71**:1263–9.

Redd WH, Montgomery GH, DuHamel KN (2001). Behavioral intervention for cancer treatment side effects. *J Nat Cancer Inst* **93**:810–23.

Richardson JL, Shelton DR, Krailo M, Levine AM (1990). The effect of compliance with treatment on survival among patients with hematologic malignancies. *J Clin Oncol* **8**:356–64

Sheard T, Maguire P (1999). The effect of psychological interventions on anxiety and depression in cancer patients: results of two meta-analyses. *Br J Cancer*, **80**:1770–80.

Slevin ML, Nichols SE, Downer SM, Wilson P, Lister TA, Arnott S *et al.* (1996). Emotional support for cancer patients: what do patients really want? *Br J Cancer* **74**:1275–9.

Smith MC, Holcome JK, Stullenbarger E (1994). A meta-analysis of intervention effectiveness for symptom management in oncology nursing research. *Oncol Nursing Forum* **21**:1201–10.

Spiegel D, Bloom JR, Yalom I (1981). Group support for patients with metastatic cancer. A randomized outcome study. *Arch Gen Psychiat* **38**:527–33.

Thorpe, R. (1998). *Patient and user perceptions of cancer care in Kingston-upon-Hull and the East Riding.* Kingston-upon-Hull: Cancer Services Project, East Riding Cancer Services Alliance.

Townsend P, Phillimore P, Beattie A (1988). *Health and deprivation. Inequality and the North.* London: Croon Helm.

Walker LG (1996). Communication skills: when, not if, to teach. *Eur J Cancer* **32A**:1457–9.

Walker LG, Anderson J (1999). Testing complementary and alternative medicine within a research protocol. *Eur J Cancer* **35**:1614–18.

Walker LG, Wesnes KA, Heys SD, Walker MB, Lolley J, Eremin O (1996). The cognitive effects of recombinant interleukin-2 (rIL-2) therapy: a controlled clinical trial using computerised assessments. *Eur J Cancer* **32A**:2275–83.

Walker LG, Walker MB, Heys SD, Lolley J, Wesnes K, Eremin O (1997). The psychological and psychiatric effects of rIL-2: a controlled clinical trial. *Psycho-Oncology* **6**:290–301.

Walker LG, Walker MB, Heys SD, Ogston K, Miller I, Hutcheon AW *et al.* (1999a). The psychological, clinical and pathological effects of relaxation training and imagery during primary chemotherapy. *Br J Cancer* **80**:262–8.

Walker LG, Heys SD, Walker MB, Ogston K, Miller I, Hutcheon AW *et al.* (1999b). Psychological factors can predict the response to primary chemotherapy in women with locally advanced breast cancer. *Eur J Cancer* **35**:1783–8.

Watson M, Denton S, Baum M, Greer S (1998). Counselling breast cancer patients: a specialist nurse service. *Counselling Psychol Quart* **1**:25–34.

Wilkinson S (1995). The changing pressures for cancer nurses 1986–93. *Eur J Cancer Care* **4**:69–74.

Williams ERL, Ramirez AJ, Richards MA, Young T, Maher EJ, Boudioni M *et al.* (2000). Are men missing from cancer information and support services? *Psycho-Oncology* **9**:364.

Worden JW, Weisman AD (1984). Preventive psychosocial intervention with newly diagnosed cancer patients. *Gen Hosp Psychiat* **6**:243–9.

Zabora J, Brintzenhofenszoc K, Curbow B, Hooker C, Piantadosi S (2001). The prevalence of psychological distress by cancer site. *Psycho-oncology* **10**:19–28.

Zigmond, AS, Snaith RT (1983). The hospital anxiety and depression scale. *Acta Psychiat Scand* **67**:361–370.

Chapter 5

Anxiety and adjustment disorders

Steven D Passik and Kenneth L Kirsh

Introduction

The many modern advances in oncology are making cancer a survivable, chronic, life-threatening illness for many patients (Bishop 1994; Brannon and Feist 1997; Passik *et al.* 1998). However, cancer is still a high magnitude stressor and patients experience, at times, catastrophic levels of stress when confronting the disease and its treatment. How a patient adapts to cancer and its accompanying treatments is key to their ongoing quality of life. Moreover, stress can have negative consequences for both physical and mental health. Accordingly, the quality of life of those living with the disease long term has become a focus of cancer care and research.

It is clear that this inherent stress takes a toll on the lives of cancer patients and their families. In a landmark study of cancer patients, Derogatis *et al.* (1983) found that the prevalence of patients having a psychiatric diagnosis was almost 50 per cent. This is a much greater percentage than the number of individuals with any psychiatric condition found in the general adult population (22 per cent) (Regier *et al.* 1993), which marks this group as being clearly at risk. Indeed, comorbidity of psychiatric diagnosis and cancer diagnosis should be viewed as the rule rather than the exception.

Psychological distress

Cancer patients have a high rate of psychiatric comorbidity. Generally, the psychological complications take the form of adjustment issues, depressed mood, anxiety, impoverished life satisfaction, or loss of self-esteem (Freidenbergs and Kaplan 1993; Molassiotis *et al.* 1995; Sarafino 1984) (see Table 5.1 for overview). However, the making of psychiatric diagnoses and the rapid identification of patients in need of help are difficult for many reasons. One problem is that psychiatric symptomatology may be mimicked by the side-effects of medication or the disease process itself in people with cancer. The shortage of time and emphasis on the physical condition alone during out-patient consultation reinforce the patients' reluctance to report psychosocial problems and can act as barriers to the recognition of psychosocial problems.

Table 5.1 Key components of the diagnoses of major depression, anxiety disorder, and adjustment disorder

Variable	Major depression	Generalized anxiety disorder	Adjustment disorder
Time course for consideration of the diagnosis	At least 2 weeks of depressed mood or anhedonia	Anxiety occurring most days for at least 6 months	Symptoms must occur within 3 months of a triggering stressor
Major features	There must be some change in either appetite, concentration, weight, sleep, feelings of guilt, suicidal ideation, or psychomotor activity. Must affect either social, occupational, or other important areas of functioning	Excessive worry and anxiety that occurs more days than not. Person reports that they have difficulty controlling the anxious feelings. Symptoms typically include either restlessness, diminished concentration, fatigue, poor sleep, muscle tension, or irritability	Marked by clinically relevant behavioural or emotional symptoms in response to an identified psychosocial stressor. Reaction causes significant impairment of social or occupational functioning. Stressor can be continuous, creating a chronic adjustment disorder
Rule-out considerations	Medication and drug side-effects. Bereavement	Medication and drug side-effects	All other major psychiatric disorders, including major depression and anxiety disorder. Bereavement
Gender prevalence	Depression is twice as common in women as in men	Approximately 60% of all cases are women, 40% are men	Men and women are equally affected

Generalized anxiety disorder

Case study

Alice was a 63-year-old retired teacher—her husband died suddenly 10 years ago and they had no children. Since taking early retirement six years ago, she had kept herself busy as a school governor and active member of her church and local community. She had very little time for herself and did not really take much notice of her swollen abdomen until she started to pass blood vaginally. A visit to the general practitioner (GP) confirmed a pelvic mass and referral to a gynaecologist for ultrasound of the abdomen confirmed a large ovarian mass. At laparotomy this was found to be stage 4 cancer of the ovary with disease extending to the omentum and multiple nodes were also discovered. Alice initially took the news in her stride accepting that she had a terminal illness. Once discharged from hospital she stayed with a friend for three weeks before returning to her own home.

Two days after returning home, she felt increasingly agitated and could not sleep or concentrate. She started telephoning her neighbours every hour expressing concern that something awful was about to happen and could not go to bed, as she was terrified that she would die during the night. She stopped eating and started to lose weight dramatically.

Eventually she was persuaded by a friend to go to the GP—she was agitated, pacing around the room tearful and distressed, and looked nearer 93 than 63. She told the GP that all she could think about was the cancer and how it was taking her over—she denied she was frightened but admitted that she was afraid to sleep.

The above case history shows how patients may present with a complex mixture of physical and psychological symptoms in the context of their frightening reality of having a diagnosis of advanced cancer. Thus the recognition of anxiety symptoms requiring treatment can be challenging. Patients with anxiety complain of tension or restlessness, or they exhibit jitteriness, autonomic hyperactivity, vigilance, insomnia, distractibility, shortness of breath, numbness, apprehension, worry, or rumination. Often the physical or somatic manifestations of anxiety overshadow the psychological or cognitive ones (Holland 1989). It is always worth considering medical causes in patients who present with anxiety, for example, uncontrolled pain, thyrotoxicosis, or alcohol or benzodiazepine withdrawl. These symptoms are a cue to further inquiry about the patient's psychological state, which is commonly one of fear, worry, or apprehension regarding the future. Anxious patients, like depressed patients, tend to selectively remember the more 'threatening information' given to them and often the process of explanation can be therapeutic in itself. In deciding whether to treat anxiety, the patient's subjective level of distress is the primary impetus for the initiation of treatment as opposed to the patient qualifying strictly for a psychiatric diagnosis. Other considerations include problematic patient behaviour such as non-compliance, family and staff reactions to the patient's distress, and the balancing of the risks and benefits of treatment (Massie 1989).

Despite the fact that anxiety in patients with advanced cancer commonly results from medical complications, it is equally often related to psychological factors related to existential issues, particularly in patients who are alert and not confused (Holland 1989). Patients frequently fear isolation and estrangement from others and may have a general sense of feeling like an outcast, Fig. 5.1. Also, financial burdens and family role changes are common stressors.

Treatment of anxiety disorders

Prevention is always better than cure—much anxiety could be prevented by better organization of services for patients with cancer. Informing patients of the results of investigations as soon as possible, ensuring that all information is communicated between primary and secondary care, and ensuring that those caring for patients with cancer possess good communication skills can all minimize morbidity. The treatment of anxiety in cancer patients involves a combination of psychotherapy and a range

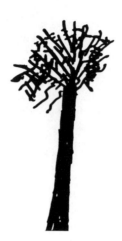

Fig. 5.1 Anxiety-Isolation.

of anxiolytic medications. The pharmacotherapy of anxiety in patients with more advanced illness involves the judicious use of the following classes of medications: benzodiazepines, neuroleptics, anti-histamines, and anti-depressants (Holland 1989; Massie 1989).

Benzodiazepines

Benzodiazepines are the mainstay of the pharmacological treatment of anxiety in cancer patients. The shorter acting benzodiazepines, such as lorazepam, alprazolam, and oxazepam, are safest in this population. The selection of these drugs avoids toxic accumulation due to impaired metabolism in debilitated individuals (Hollister 1986). Lorazepam and oxazepam are metabolized by conjugation in the liver and are there-fore safest in patients with hepatic disease. This is in contrast to alprazolam and other benzodiazepines that are metabolized through oxidative pathways in the liver that are more vulnerable to interference with hepatic damage. The disadvantage of using short-acting benzodiazepines is that patients often experience breakthrough anxiety or end-of-dose distress. Such patients can benefit from switching to longer acting benzodiazepines such as diazepam or clonazepam. Common dosage regimens include lorazepam at 0.5–2.0 mg (as required), diazepam at 2.5–10 mg (as required), and clonazepam at 1–2 mg. Clonazepam has been found to be extremely useful, in our setting, for the treatment of symptoms of anxiety. Patients who experience end-of-dose failure with recurrence of anxiety on shorter acting drugs also find clonazepam helpful. Clonazepam is also useful in patients with organic mood disorders who have symptoms of mania and as an adjuvant analgesic in patients with neuropathic pain (Chouinard *et al.* 1983; Walsh 1990). Fears of causing respiratory depression should not prevent the clinician from using adequate dosages of benzodiazepines to control anxiety. The likelihood of respiratory depression is minimized when shorter acting drugs are prescribed and the drug dosages are increased in small increments.

Non-benzodiazepine anxiolytics

Typical and atypical neuroleptics, such as thioridazine, haloperidol, and olanzapine are useful in the treatment of anxiety when benzodiazepines are not sufficient for symptom control. They are also indicated when an organic aetiology is suspected or when psychotic symptoms such as delusions or hallucinations accompany the anxiety. Typically, haloperidol at 0.5–3 mg (as required) is sufficient to control symptoms of anxiety and avoid excessive sedation. Low potency neuroleptics such as thioridazine are effective anxiolytics which can help with insomnia and agitation (thioridazine, although widely available in Europe and the USA, is currently unavailable in the UK). The atypical neuroleptics, such as olanzapine, can control anxiety related to confusional states, delusions, and nausea (Passik and Cooper 1999). Neuroleptics are perhaps the safest class of anxiolytics in patients where there is legitimate concern regarding respiratory depression or compromise. Methotrimeprazine is a phenothiazine with anxiolytic properties that is often used for the treatment of pain and anxiety in the patient with advanced cancer (Oliver 1985). Its side-effects include sedation, anti-cholinergic symptoms, and hypotension. It can be useful in patients where sedation is desirable. With this class of drugs in general, one must be aware of extrapyramidal side-effects (particularly when patients are taking additional neuroleptics for antiemetic purposes) and the remote possibility of neuroleptic malignant syndrome. Tardive dyskinesia is rarely a concern given the generally short-term usage and low dosages of these medications in this population (Breitbart 1986).

Tricyclic, selective serotonin reuptake inhibitors (SSRI), and heterocyclic antidepressants are the most effective treatment for anxiety accompanying depression and are helpful in treating panic disorder (Liebowitz 1985; Popkin et al. 1985). Our research (Theobald et al. in press) has shown that mirtazapine is particularly useful for this use in cancer populations.

Buspirone is a non-benzodiazepine anxiolytic that is useful along with psychotherapy in patients with chronic anxiety or anxiety related to adjustment disorders. The onset of anxiolytic action is delayed in comparison to the benzodiazepines, taking five to 10 days for relief of anxiety to begin. Since buspirone is not a benzodiazepine, it will not block benzodiazepine withdrawal, and so one must be cautious when switching from a benzodiazepine to buspirone. Due to its delayed onset of action and indication for use in chronic anxiety states, buspirone may have limited usefulness to the clinician treating anxiety in the rehabilitation setting with cancer patients.

Non-pharmacological treatment of anxiety disorders

Non-pharmacological interventions for anxiety and distress include supportive psychotherapy and behavioural interventions, which are used alone or in combination. Brief supportive psychotherapy is often useful in dealing with both crisis-related issues as well as existential issues (Massie et al. 1989). Psychotherapeutic interventions often include both the patient and family, particularly as the patient with cancer becomes increasingly debilitated and less able to interact. The goals of psychotherapy for the anxious patient are to establish a bond that decreases the sense of isolation; to help the patient face cancer with a sense of integrity and self worth; to correct misconceptions about the past and present; to integrate the present illness into a continuum of life experiences; and to explore issues of separation, loss, and the unknown that lies ahead.

Complementary therapies such as aromatherapy and massage and specific interventions such as hypnosis, relaxation, and imagery may help reduce anxiety and thereby increase the patient's sense of control. Most patients with cancer, even those with advanced disease, are appropriate candidates for useful application of behavioural techniques despite physical debilitation. In assessing the utility of such interventions for a given patient, the clinician should take into account the patient's mental clarity. Confusional states interfere dramatically with a patient's ability to focus attention and thus limit the usefulness of these techniques (Breitbart 1989). A typical behavioural intervention for anxiety includes a relaxation exercise combined with some distraction or imagery technique. The patient is first taught to relax with passive breathing accompanied by either passive or active muscle relaxation. Once in such a relaxed state, the patient is taught a pleasant, distracting imagery exercise. In a randomized study comparing a relaxation technique with alprazolam in the treatment of anxiety and distress in cancer patients, both treatments were demonstrated to be quite effective for mild to moderate degrees of anxiety or distress. The drug intervention (alprazolam) was more effective for greater levels of distress or anxiety and had more rapid onset of beneficial effect (Adams *et al.* 1986). Often, such interventions are used in combination, for example, utilizing relaxation techniques concurrently with anxiolytic medications in highly anxious cancer patients.

Anxiety and agitation during the last few weeks and days of life is distressing for the patient, relatives, and staff. Even the very ill patient can derive great benefit from being encouraged to share their fears and anxieties with others. At this stage there may be concerns over previous experiences or rifts in the family and a visit from a family member who has not visited for months or even years is often found to ease the distress.

Sedation either orally or subcutaneously with a benzodiazepine (for example, midazolam) can calm the patient whilst still allowing them to work through some of these issues.

Adjustment disorder—definition

Adjustment disorder, according to the fourth edition of the *Diagnostic and statistical manual of mental disorders* (*DSM-IV*) (American Psychiatric Association 1994), is a rather nebulous disorder characterized by a variety of clinically significant behavioural or emotional symptoms that occur as a result of some triggering event or stressor. For diagnostic purposes there can also be a mixture of the aforementioned subtypes or the disorder may remain unspecified when the symptoms cannot be clearly classified. The onset of adjustment disorder must occur within three months of the triggering event and it must not continue longer than six months after the termination of the stressor or its consequences. However, the disorder can be deemed to be chronic, thus lasting more than six months, when there is a chronic stressor or when the consequences of the stressor have long-term impact, for example, advanced cancer. Finally, adjustment disorder can only be diagnosed if the disturbance is identifiable and does not meet the criteria for other identifiable psychiatric disorders, such as major depression or generalized anxiety disorder, and if the symptoms are not a result of bereavement.

The *International classification of disease-10* (World Health Organization 1995) also has a similar diagnosis for adjustment disorder, with a few minor exceptions. First, the reaction to the stressor has to occur within a one-month span of time. Second, the subtypes are different and are labelled separately with names such as brief depressive reaction and disturbance of emotions and conduct. Finally, one of the subtypes, prolonged depressive reaction, may last for up to two years. Thus, while the disorder is little understood, and some claim that it does not exist (Depue and Monroe 1986; Vinokur and Caplan 1986), there is at least a global attempt to explain the phenomenon.

Differential diagnosis of adjustment disorder

Adjustment disorder is the most prevalent problem associated with cancer. In fact, it is evident in 25–30% of all patients with cancer (Derogatis *et al.* 1983; Dugan *et al.* 1998). Despite this high prevalence, most efforts at screening for psychiatric problems in patients with cancer have focused on major depression rather than so-called minor depression, or adjustment disorder. Moreover, as mentioned earlier, genuine problems in adjustment can be obscured by organic effects of cancer and cancer treatment. Certain drugs used in the treatment of cancer, such as prednisolone, procarbazine, vinicristine, and vinblastine cause depressive symptoms that may be confused with adjustment disorder or mood disorder through their side-effects. Such confounding of the diagnosis can lead to inadequate treatment being offered to patients or cause the disorder to be overlooked or explained as a probable drug side-effect.

Adjustment disorder and depression

The relationship between adjustment disorder and major depression may be explained from two main viewpoints. First, one may speculate that adjustment disorder is simply quantitatively different from major depression. This is the notion that mood disorders and adjustment disorders lie along a continuum and the main differentiation is one of severity (Angst and Dobler-Mikola 1984). This conceptualization as a 'subclinical depression' leads to an approach whereby moderate scores on traditional depression screens are thought to be diagnostic for this disorder (Strain 1998). However, there is no uniform agreement on what cut-offs should be used, if indeed it is a minor or subclinical depression. In other words, adjustment disorder may occupy a niche role somewhere between a major depressive disorder and the normal unhappiness experienced under extreme stress (Depression Guideline Panel 1993).

An alternative conceptualization of the relationship between adjustment disorder and major depressive disorder is that the two disorders are qualitatively or categorically distinct. According to this point of view, major depression is seen as a symptom-based diagnosis (for example, anhedonia for more than two weeks) whereas adjustment disorder is more function based (for example, inability to maintain role functioning).

A recent study (Passik *et al.* 2001) shows that a traditional depression screen does not adequately identify adjustment disorder in ambulatory oncology patients.

Adjustment disorder diagnosis as a marker of psychological distress

The underdiagnosis and undertreatment of psychological problems in patients with advanced cancer, and subsequent negative impact in quality of life, remain highly prevalent (Dugan *et al.* 1998; Katon and Sullivan 1990; Zabora 1998). It is clear that people with psychological distress in general and adjustment disorder in particular are not being diagnosed or recognized by oncology professionals (Razavi *et al.* 1990).

In a drive to address this large problem, Holland (1997) has called for a major goal of psycho-oncology to be that all patient distress is recognized and treated. In a similar vein, the National Comprehensive Cancer Network (NCCN) has also acknowledged that a crisis is developing regarding the lack of psychosocial screening for distress (American Society of Psychosocial and Behavioral Oncology/Aids 1999). Although using the term 'distress' to avoid perceived stigma by patients, the NCCN defines it as an unpleasant emotional experience of a social or psychological nature that is tied to and interferes with the ability to effectively cope with cancer and cancer-related treatment. The NCCN further state that there are no standards of care for the psychosocial domain of cancer care and that there is no referral pattern or algorithm for identifying the level of distress or appropriate treatment modalities. Finally, as a way to remedy the situation, they are calling for the development or identification of rapid, brief screening tools that can measure distress in clinics and that can be administered by the oncology or palliative care team. The use of such tools should be carried out with respect to their psychometric qualities and relationship to clinical diagnoses.

Identification of adjustment disorder

The identification and diagnosis of adjustment disorder is not straightforward. One of the problems with the adjustment disorder diagnosis is that it lacks precise features. The first problem comes in discussing the stressor or triggering event. There are no guidelines or criteria in the *DSM-IV* for quantifying the stressors leading to adjustment disorder in a given individual (Zilberg *et al.* 1982). It is also difficult to define accurately what constitutes maladaptive behaviour especially under circumstances of monumental stress. There are no universal guidelines and the subjective severity of symptoms or decrement in social function can vary widely within a given individual (Fabrega *et al.* 1987).

There is no doubt that overlap exists between the disorders of major depression, generalized anxiety disorder, and adjustment disorder. However, the diagnosis of adjustment disorder requires that the patient does not qualify for these other diagnoses. Therefore, they can qualify for the diagnosis only if they manifest problems of adapting to the stressor but do not meet criteria for these other diagnoses. The challenge this poses to screening is that there is a need to identify key areas that separate adjustment disorder from major depression in terms of detection. To this end, the notion of coping inflexibility in response to the illness or treatment has been suggested.

It is believed that one of the personality factors that may lead to problems of adjustment is a lack of coping flexibility on the part of the patient regarding illness and illness-related treatment (Carson *et al.* 1989; Rogers and LeUnes 1979). Those who develop adjustment disorder may be more likely to be rigid in their thinking and determined to address new problems in the manner they did prior to the onset of illness. If the prior coping and problem-solving strategies fail, the person may begin to exhibit the emotional reactions (depressed mood and anxiety) associated with adjustment disorder, in contrast to those who have an adaptive style that focuses on being flexible (Lee 1983). This concept has never been formally operationalized for use in assessment and detecting adjustment disorder in cancer patients. Further, there is increasing recognition that a lack of effective, flexible coping is prevalent in cancer patients in distress and that this lack of flexible coping is not being recognized (American Society of Psychosocial and Behavioral Oncology/Aids 1999).

We conducted a study on the identification of adjustment disorders. The study was specifically an attempt to explore issues related to screening for adjustment disorder. Commonly used scales for depression, anxiety, and quality of life along with two pilot tools were employed for the purpose of detecting patients with psychological distress who met criteria for a diagnosis of adjustment disorder as determined by the structured clinical interview for *DSM-IV* (SCID). Two novel instruments were introduced and piloted during the study to gather initial data and suggestions for items to be included on potential screening tools to undergo a future full psychometric exploration. Both measures exhibited good reliability and overall psychometric properties.

The study results offered some interesting findings. First, none of the scales were significant predictors of adjustment disorder on the SCID, although many were able to detect general distress as defined by the presence of any psychological disorder. Thus, a quick and easy method for detecting adjustment disorder remained elusive. Second, having any mental illness (or psychiatric) diagnosis was a good predictor of reduced quality of life. Third, quality of life impact varied with psychiatric diagnosis. Participants with adjustment disorder had significantly higher quality of life ratings than the comparison group of participants with either major depression or anxiety, although lower quality of life than those with no psychiatric diagnosis. This provides some initial evidence that, compared to other psychiatric diagnoses or to the absence of psychiatric diagnosis, adjustment disorder may be useful as an independent and identifiable disorder as postulated earlier, with implications for quality of life and well-being that are both different from and less severe than for other psychiatric disorders.

Treatment of adjustment disorder

Patients identified as having adjustment disorder are often associated with being at risk for increased morbidity and even mortality (that is, suicide) (DeLeo *et al.* 1986). It is important to note, however, that people with adjustment disorder have been shown to have positive outcomes when they are treated with brief psychotherapy (Sifneos 1989), the usual form of psychotherapy employed by psycho-oncologists. This allows for the possibility of early treatment delivered by nurse specialists and other staff before a problem worsens to the point of requiring more intensive care and medications (Miller 1996; Samuelian *et al.* 1994; Snyder *et al.* 1990). Psychotherapy for adjustment disorder addresses the stressors directly by teaching enhanced coping skills and is focused on immediacy. Establishing social support networks and psychoeducation is also employed (Pollin and Holland 1992; Wise 1994). Informal support groups and more formal group therapy have been shown to be highly effective for improving quality of life and decreasing depression and anxiety symptoms in cancer patients (Spiegel 1981; Zabora 1998). The rapid identification of adjustment disorder can prompt early psychological intervention that can help to promote the patient's quality of life, or at the very least, may prevent the further erosion of the patient's ability to function.

Advanced cancer patients with depressive symptomatology are often reacting to the burden of the illness and the effect it has on their lives. Clinicians working in oncology rely primarily on short-term supportive psychotherapy based on a crisis intervention model to help patients with depressive symptoms. Cognitive–behavioural techniques are often integrated into treatment and are very useful and effective. These therapies explore methods of enhancing coping and problem-solving skills, facilitating communication between the patient and others, revitalizing social support networks, and reshaping negative or self-defeating thoughts. The treating clinician should be aware that a number of factors will influence the individual patient's reaction to the disease— medical factors, such as the site and clinical course of the disease along with the type of treatment received; psychological factors, such as adjustment to prior illnesses and losses, concurrent life stresses, family history of depression and suicide, and developmental life phase; and social factors, such as availability of support from family, friends, and coworkers—and that these will affect the patients' ability to adjust.

The crisis intervention model is the basis for much oncology-related psychotherapy. Crisis intervention is a process for actively influencing psychosocial functioning during a period of disequilibrium. It is directed at alleviating the immediate impact of disruptive stressful events. The aim is to reduce emotional distress while working toward strengthening the patient's psychological and social resources. Generally, crisis therapy is time limited and asserts clear-cut goals (Parad and Parad 1990). Supportive crisis intervention psychotherapy involves clarifying information and answering questions about the illness and its treatment, correcting misunderstanding, and giving reassurance about the situation. Describing common reactions to illness may help the patient and their family to normalize their experience. Patients' usual adaptive strategies should be explored and their strengths supported as needed in adjustment. The patients should be encouraged to discuss how they feel about their lifestyle modifications, their family role changes, and their fears of dependency and abandonment. Themes of loss and anticipatory grief can be useful to discuss. The patients often experience loss of good health, loss of body integrity, loss of self-esteem, along with losses secondary to cancer (for example, financial, social, and occupational). Therapy should improve a sense of control and morale. When the focus of treatment changes from cure to palliation, it will be extremely important for the patient to know that while curative treatment has ended they will not be abandoned and that their comfort, pain control, and dignity will receive continued attention.

Cognitive–behavioural interventions help patients allay exaggerated fears by encouraging them to consider different possible outcomes for their situation. Helping patients focus on what aspects of the disease and its treatment they have control over and encouraging behaviour modification that will keep them involved and positive could provide a better quality of life for these patients. Relaxation techniques and imagery may enhance any of these therapeutic interventions. Simple focused breathing exercises, meditation, and progressive muscle relaxation can be used to lessen episodic anxiety that many cancer patients experience. Pleasant imagery, such as visualizing a gentle stream flowing through a beautiful landscape, can also ease tension some patients feel.

Self-help groups and hospice day care are useful interventions for cancer patients and family members who are distressed. The professionally run groups will usually use educational, supportive, or cognitive–behavioural methods while the lay groups generally focus on education, practical advice, modelling, and serving as a source of mutual support and advocacy.

Conclusions

Patients with advanced cancer often have comorbid psychiatric problems including a high frequency of adjustment disorders and anxiety. The identification and management of these disorders can often be accomplished by the oncology staff but the provision of appropriate mental health staff, for example, those involved in social work, liaison psychiatry, and psychology is invaluable. Working together, the team can enhance quality of life for the patient and family.

References

Adams F, Fernandez F, Andersson B (1986). Emergency pharmacotherapy of delirium in the critically ill cancer patient. *Psychosomatics* **27**:33–7.

American Psychiatric Association (1994). *Diagnostic and statistical manual of mental disorders.* 4th edn. Washington, DC: American Psychiatric Association.

American Society of Psychosocial and Behavioral Oncology/AIDS (1999). *Standards of care for the management of distress in patients with cancer.* New York: American Society of Psychosocial and Behavioral Oncology/AIDS.

Angst J, Dobler-Mikola A (1984). The Zurich study II: The continuum from normal to pathological depressive mood swings. *Eur Arch Psych Neurol Sci* **234**:21–9.

Bishop G (1994). *Health psychology: integrating mind and body.* Boston: Allyn and Bacon.

Brannon L, Feist J (1997). *Health psychology: An introduction to behavior and health.* Boston: Brooks/Cole.

Breitbart W (1986). Tardive dyskinesia associated with high dose intravenous metaclopramide. *N Eng J Med* **315**:518–19.

Breitbart W (1989). Psychiatric management of cancer pain. *Cancer* **63**:2336–42.

Carson D, Council J, Volk M (1989). Temperament as a predictor of psychological adjustment in female adult incest victims. *J Clin Psychiat* **452**:330–5.

Chouinard G, Young S, Annable L (1983). Antimanic effect of clonazepam. *Biol Psychiat* **18**:451–66.

DeLeo D, Pellagrin C, Cerate L (1986). Adjustment disorders and suicidality. *Psychiat Rep* **59:**355–8.

Depression Guideline Panel (1993). Depression in primary care: Volume 1. Detection and diagnosis. Clinical practice guideline No. 5. Rockville, MD: US Department of Health and Human Services, Public Health Service, Agency for Health Care Policy and Research, AHPCR. Publication No. 93–0550.

Depue R, Monroe S (1986). Conceptualization and measurement of human disorder in life stress research: The problem of chronic disturbance. *Psychiat Bul* **99:**36–51.

Derogatis L, Morrow G, Fetting J (1983). The prevalence of psychiatric disorders among cancer patients. *JAMA* **249:**751–7.

Dugan W, McDonald M, Passik S, Rosenfeld B, Theobald D, Edgerton S (1998). Use of the Zung self-rating depression scale in cancer patients: feasibility as a screening tool. *Psycho-oncology* **7:**483–93.

Fabrega H, Mezzich J, Mezzich A (1987). Adjustment disorder as a marginal or transitional illness category in DSM-III. *Arch Gen Psychiat* **44:**567–72.

Friedenbergs I, Kaplan E (1993). Cancer. In: Eisenberg M, Glueckauf R, Zaretsky H (ed.). *Medical aspects of disability: a handbook for the rehabilitation professional.* New York: Springer. pp. 105–18.

Holland J (1989). Anxiety and cancer: the patient and family. *J Clin Psychiat* **50:**20–5.

Holland J (1997). Preliminary guidelines for the treatment of distress. *Oncology* **11:**109–14.

Hollister L (1986). Pharmacotherapeutic considerations in anxiety disorders. *J Clin Psychiat* **47:**33–6.

Katon W, Sullivan M (1990). Depression and chronic medical illness. *J Clin Psychiat* **51 (suppl 6):**3–11.

Lee R (1983). Returning to work: potential problems for mid-career mothers. *J Sex Marital Ther* **9:**219–32.

Liebowtiz M (1985). Imipramine in the treatment of panic disorder and its complications. *Psychiat Clin North Am* **8:**37–47.

Massie M (1989). Anxiety, panic and phobias. In: Holland J, Rowland J. (ed.). *Handbook of Psychooncology: psychological care of the patient with cancer.* New York: Oxford University Press. pp. 300–9.

Massie M, Holland J, Straker N (1989). Psychotherapeutic interventions. In: Holland JC, Rowland JH (ed.). *Handbook of psychooncology: psychological care of the patient with cancer.* New York: Oxford University Press. pp. 455–69.

Miller J (1996). Adjustment disorder. [On-line]. Available at: www.athealth.com.

Molassiotis A, Boughton B, Burgoyne T, Van den Akker O (1995). Comparison of the overall quality of life in 50 long-term survivors of autologous and allogeneic bone marrow transplantation. *J Adv Nursing* **22:**509–16.

Oliver D (1985). The use of methotrimeprazine in terminal care. *Br J Clin Pract* **39:**339–40.

Parad HJ, Parad LG (1990). Crisis intervention: an introductory overview. In: Parad HJ, Parad LG (ed.). *Crisis intervention: the practitioner's sourcebook for brief therapy.* Wisconsin: Family Service America. pp. 3–68.

Passik S, Cooper M (1999). Complicated delirium in a cancer patient successfully treated with olanzapine. *J Pain Sympt Management* **17:**219–23.

Passik S, Kirsh K, Donaghy K, Theobald D, Lundberg J, Lundberg E (2001). An attempt to employ the Zung self-rating depression scale as a lab test to trigger follow-up in ambulatory oncology clinics: criterion validity and detection. *J Pain Sympt Management* **21**:273–81.

Passik S, Dugan W, McDonald M, Rosenfeld B, Theobald D, Edgerton S (1998). Oncologists' recognition of depression in their patients with cancer. *J Clin Oncol* **16**:1594–1600.

Pollin I, Holland J (1992). A model for counseling the medically ill: the Linda Pollin Foundation Approach. *Gen Hosp Psychiat* **14**:11–24.

Popkin M, Callies A, Mackenzie T (1985). The outcome of antidepressant use in the medically ill. *Arch Gen Psychiat* **42**:1160–3.

Razavi D, Delvaux N, Farvacques C (1990). Screening for adjustment disorders and major depressive disorders in cancer patients. *Br J Psychiat* **156**:79–83.

Regier D, Narrow W, Rae D (1993). The *de facto* mental and addictive disorders service system. Epidemiologic catchement area prospective 1-year prevalence rates of disorders and services. *Arch Gen Psychiat* **50**:85–94.

Rogers S, LeUnes A (1979). A psychometric and behavioral comparison of delinquents who were abused as children with their non-abused peers. *J Clin Psychiat* **35**:470–2.

Samuelian J, Charlot V, Derynck F, Rouillon F (1994). Adjustment disorders. Apropos of an epidemiologic survey. *Encephale* **20**(6):755–65.

Sarafino E (1994). *Health psychology: biopsychosocial interactions*. 2nd edn. New York: John Wiley.

Sifneos P (1989). Brief dynamic and crisis therapy. In: Kaplan H, Sadock B. (ed.). *Comprehensive textbook of psychiatry, Vol. 2*. 5th edn. Baltimore: Williams & Wilkins. pp. 1562–7.

Snyder S, Strain J, Wolf D (1990). Differentiating major depression from adjustment disorder with depressed mood in the medical setting. *Gen Hosp Psych* **12**(3):159–65.

Spiegel D (1981). Group support for patients with metastatic cancer. A randomized outcome study. *Arch Gen Psychiat* **38**:527–33.

Strain J (1998). Adjustment disorders. In: Holland J. (ed.). *Psycho-oncology*. New York: Oxford University Press. pp. 509–17.

Theobald DE, Kirsh KL, Holtsclaw E, Donaghy K, Passik SD (in press). An open label crossover trial of mirtazapine (15 and 30 mg) in cancer patients with pain and other distressing symptoms. *J Pain Sympt Managment*.

Vinokur A, Caplan R (1986). Cognitive and affective components of life events. Their relations and effects on well-being. *Am J Community Psychiat* **14**:351–71.

Walsh T (1990). Adjuvant analgesic therapy in cancer pain. In: Foley KM, Bonica JJ, Ventafridda. J (ed.). *Advances in pain research and therapy, Vol. 16, Second International Congress on Cancer Pain*. New York: Raven Press. pp. 155–66.

Wise M (1994). Adjustment disorders and impulse disorders not otherwise classified. In: Talbot J, Hales R, Yudofsky S (ed.). *The American psychiatric press textbook of psychiatry*. 2nd edn. Washington, DC: American Psychiatric Press, pp. 211–23.

World Health Organization (1995). *International classification of diseases*. 10th edn. Geneva: World Health Organization.

Zabora J (1998). Screening procedures for psychosocial distress. In: Holland J. (ed.). *Psycho-oncology*. New York: Oxford University Press. pp. 653–61.

Zilberg N, Weiss D, Horowitz M (1982). Impact of event scales: cross-validation study and some empirical evidence supporting a conceptual model of stress response syndromes. *J Consult Clin Psychiat* **50**:407–14.

Chapter 6

Diagnosis, assessment, and treatment of depression in palliative care

Hayley Pessin, Mordecai Potash, and William Breitbart

Introduction

Recent advances in palliative care highlight the importance of expanding our concepts of adequate palliative care, beyond a focus on pain and physical symptom control, to include psychiatric, psychosocial, existential, and spiritual domains of care. Therefore, skills in diagnostic assessment of psychiatric disorders in patients with terminal cancer are of increasing importance to palliative care practitioners. The diagnosis and management of depression in patients with advanced cancer is perhaps the most difficult and important psychiatric issue confronting palliative care practitioners.

A number of medical and psychosocial issues such as medication side-effects, physical impairments, dependency, loss of autonomy, anticipatory grief, and family dysfunction, all of which frequently co-occur during a terminal illness, can increase the risk of psychological distress and depressive symptomatology at the end of life (Breitbart *et al.* 1998). Depressed mood and sadness are common, even appropriate responses, for patients who are facing a terminal illness (Plate 3, pp. 98–99). Yet, despite the common occurrence of feelings of sadness and depression among terminally ill individuals, these symptoms, although often ameliorable, frequently remain unrecognized and untreated, as they are dismissed as 'normal reactions' even in the face of severe affective disturbance. This chapter reviews the prevalence, risk factors, assessment, and management of depression in terminally ill cancer patients. It will provide the tools to effectively recognize, address, and care for patients experiencing depression at the end of life in order to minimize distress and offer a more comprehensive approach to palliative care.

Prevalence of depression in palliative care

A number of studies have examined the prevalence of major depression in cancer patients with far-advanced disease (Derogatis *et al.* 1983; Kathol *et al.* 1990*a*;

Chochinov *et al.* 1994; Minagawa *et al.* 1996). These studies suggest that depression commonly occurs in later stages of cancer, ranging in prevalence from 3.2 to 52 per cent (see Table 6.1). The broad variation in the reported prevalence of depression in this population is due, in part, to the problems of terminology and methodology and the application of diagnostic systems not originally intended for use in cancer patients. In addition, differences across settings and clinical populations (for example, ambulatory, advanced cancer, or hospice patients) may contribute to wide variations across prevalence studies. Methodological issues such as the use of different diagnostic criteria represent a major source of inconsistency. Another concern is that the diagnosis of adjustment disorders is sometimes included in the prevalence study. Studies that include the diagnosis of adjustment disorders as a separate diagnosis tend to report lower rates of the more severe major depressive disorder. Finally, the sample characteristics and inclusion criteria may impact prevalence rates significantly especially at the end of life where psychiatric comorbidity is highly prevalent. Breitbart *et al.* (2000)

Table 6.1 Prevalence of depressive disorders among advanced cancer patients

Study	Population	n	Diagnostic criteria	Prevalence
Alexander *et al.* (1993)	mixed in-patients	60	*DSM-III-R*	12% major depression 2% dysthymia 17% adjustment disorder with depression
Breitbart *et al.* (2000)	mixed palliative care in-patients	92	*DSM-IV* HDRS	18% major depression
Bukberg *et al.* (1984)	mixed in-patients	62	*DSM-III* (excluded somatic symptoms)	42% major depression
Chochinov *et al.* (1995)	mixed palliative care in-patients	200	*RDC*	8% major depression 5% minor depression
Derogatis *et al.* (1983)	mixed in-patients and out-patients	215	*DSM-III*	6% major depression 12% adjustment disorder with depression
Evans *et al.* (1986)	gynaecology in-patients	83	*DSM-III*	23% major depression
Kelsen *et al.* (1995)	pancreatic cancer	130	BDI	38% major depression
Lansky *et al.* (1985)	mixed women out-patients and in-patients	505	*DSM-III*	5% major depression
Razavi *et al.* (1990)	mixed in-patients	210	Endicott criteria/*DSM-III* HADS	8% major depression 52% adjustment disorder
Minagawa *et al.* (1996)	palliative care in-patients	109	*DSM-III*	3.2% major depression 7.5% adjustment disorder

BDI, Beck depression inventory; HADS, hospital anxiety and depression scale; HDRS, Hamilton Depression Rating Scale.

excluded patients with organic mental disorders in a sample of palliative care in-patients and reported a much higher incidence of major depression (17.5 per cent).

In summary, the available literature on the prevalence of depression in advanced cancer patients suggests that the rate of depression is elevated in cancer as compared to the general population. Furthermore, even when the most stringent criteria are used, about 5–15 per cent of patients with cancer will meet criteria for major depression. Furthermore, another 10–15 per cent of patients present with symptoms that, while less severe, still require treatment. There is good empirical support for the conclusion that at least a quarter of patients with advanced cancer will present with a significant degree of dysphoria (Massie 1989). This general figure also corresponds well with perceptions of family members' reporting on the psychological well-being of their dying relatives (Lynn *et al.* 1997).

Diagnosis and assessment of depression in palliative care

Criterion-based diagnostic system

A criterion-based diagnostic system includes approaches such as the fourth edition of the *Diagnostic and statistical manual of mental disorders* (*DSM-IV*) (American Psychiatric Association 1994) or its predecessors (*DS-III* and *DSM-III-R*) and the *Research diagnostic criteria* (*RDC*) (Spitzer *et al.* 1978). These systems are based on the assumption that depression is a distinct syndromal disorder characterized by a constellation of symptoms, of a certain minimal level of severity and duration, and associated with impairment in functional and social roles. Patients are classified as having a depressive episode based on whether or not they meet these specific criteria.

The symptoms that must be assessed to make the diagnosis of depression are listed in the *DSM-IV* (see Table 6.2). Utilization of the different diagnostic classification systems, such as the *DSM-III*, *DSM-IV*, and the *RDC*), often leads to widely varying rates of detection of depression in patients with life-threatening illness. Certainly, the *DSM-IV* diagnostic criteria for depression are the most widely accepted and best-validated tool for diagnosis. Table 6.3 outlines questions used to assess symptoms of depression based on the *DSM-IV* criteria.

Diagnostic interviews

There are several different approaches to assessment procedures, which are categorized into criterion-based diagnostic systems, diagnostic interviews, and self-report measures (see Table 6.4). The focus here will be diagnostic interviews, as self-report measures are addressed more fully in the chapter on assessment. For research purposes, diagnostic assessments are usually conducted using structured interviews such as the diagnostic interview schedule (DIS) (Robins *et al.* 1981), the structured clinical interview for *DSM-III-R* (SCID) (Spitzer *et al.* 1990), or the schedule for affective disorders and schizophrenia (SADS) (Endicott and Spitzer 1978). These interviews differ with respect to their degree of structure and in the formats with which the interviewer codes the patient's verbal responses. The DIS is highly structured and designed for use

Table 6.2 *DSM-IV* criteria for major depressive syndrome

A. At least five of the following symptoms have been persistent for 2 weeks or more (at least one symptom must be (1) or (2))

  (1) depressed mood or dysphoria most of the day, nearly everyday

  (2) loss of interest or pleasure or anhedonia

  (3) sleep disorder, insomnia, or hypersomnia

  (4) appetite or weight change

  (5) fatigue or loss of energy

  (6) feelings of worthlessness or guilt

  (7) indecisiveness or poor concentration

  (8) thoughts of death or suicidal ideation

B. The symptoms do not meet criteria for a mixed episode

C. The symptoms cause clinically significant social or occupational impairment

D. The symptoms are not due to the direct physiological effects of a substance or a general medical condition

E. The symptoms are not better accounted for by bereavement

---

by lay interviewers. The SCID and SADS are semi-structured and are intended for use by clinicians. With the DIS and the SCID, the interviewer is required to code specific symptoms as being either present or absent, whereas with the SADS, the interviewer rates the severity of symptoms on ordinal scales. All of these interview protocols have been subjected to extensive checks of their reliability and validity. If administered in their entirety, these interviews cover a broad range of common mental disorders. However, they can be very time consuming, which is a serious limitation to their use in palliative care settings. More commonly, investigators administer only the modules within an interview that address depression in order to minimize patient burden. There are also a number of self-report measures that are discussed in a later chapter on screening for depression.

Issues in assessment of depression in the terminally ill

The most common diagnostic difficulty that arises in palliative care settings is how to interpret the physical or somatic symptoms patients present with in the context of a possible depression. The challenge is to determine whether these symptoms are part of the depression syndrome or a direct biological result of advancing cancer. In answering this question, five different approaches to the diagnosis of major depression in the terminally ill patient have been described (Spitzer *et al.* 1994; Breitbart *et al.* 1995). These approaches are (1) an inclusive approach, which includes all symptoms whether or not they may be secondary to illness or treatment; (2) an exclusive approach, which deletes and disregards all physical symptoms from consideration, not allowing them to contribute to a diagnosis of major depressive syndrome; (3) an aetiologic approach, in which the clinician attempts to determine whether the physical symptom is due to cancer illness or treatment (and so does not include it) or due to a depressive disorder

Table 6.3 Questions to assess depressive symptoms

Cognitive/emotional symptom questions	Symptom
How well are you coping with your cancer? Well? Poorly?	Well-being
How are your spirits since diagnosis? Down? Blue? Do you cry sometimes? How often? Only alone?	Mood
Are there things you still enjoy doing? Have you lost pleasure in things you use to do before you had cancer?	Anhedonia
How does the future look to you? Bright? Black? Do you feel you can influence your care or is your care totally under others' control?	Hopelessness
Do you worry about being a burden to family or friends during treatment for cancer?	Worthlessness
Do you feel others might be better off without you?	Guilt
Have you had any thoughts of not wanting to live or you would be better off dead?	Suicidal ideation
Have you stopped taking care of yourself or thought about hurting yourself?	Suicidal plan
Physical symptom questions	*Symptom*
Do you have pain that isn't controlled?	Pain
How much time do you spend in bed? Do you feel weak? Fatigue easily? Rested after sleep? Any relationship to change in treatment or how you feel otherwise physically?	Fatigue
How is your sleeping? Trouble going to sleep? Awake often?	Insomnia
How is your appetite? Does food taste good? Any change in weight?	Appetite
How is your interest in sex? Has there been a change in how frequently you have sex?	Libido
Do you have problems coming up with thoughts? Have you felt that your thoughts are slower than usual?	Concentration
Have you been moving more slowly than usual?	Psychomotor

(in which case it is included as a criterion symptom); (4) a high-diagnostic-threshold approach, which requires that patients have seven (instead of five) criteria symptoms for major depression; and (5) a substitutive approach, where physical symptoms of an uncertain aetiology are replaced by other non-somatic symptoms. The latter approach is best exemplified by the Endicott substitution criteria (Endicott 1984) (see Table 6.5).

While there are advantages and disadvantages to each of the approaches above, there is not a clear consensus as to which one is the best approach for accurately diagnosing depression in the terminally ill. Chochinov *et al.* (1994) studied the prevalence of depression in a terminally ill cancer population and compared low and high diagnostic thresholds, as well as Endicott substitution criteria. Interestingly, identical prevalence rates of 9.2 per cent for major depression and 3.8 per cent for minor

Table 6.4 Research assessment methods for depression in cancer patients

Criterion-based diagnostic systems

Diagnostic and statistical manual (DSM-III, III-R, IV)

Endicott substitution criteria

Research diagnostic criteria (RDC)

Structured diagnostic interviews

Schedule for affective disorders and schizophrenia (SADS)

Diagnostic interview schedule (DIS)

Structured clinical interview for *DSM-III-R* (SCID)

Primary care evaluation of mental disorders (PRIME MD)

Screening instruments—self-report

General health questionnaire-30

Hospital anxiety and depression scale (HADS)

Beck depression inventory (BDI)

Rotterdam symptom checklist (RSCL)

Carroll depression rating scale (SDRS)

Table 6.5 Endicott substitution criteria

Physical/somatic	Psychological symptom substitute
Change in appetite or weight	Tearfulness Depressed appearance
Sleep disturbance	Social withdrawal Decreased talkativeness
Fatigue or loss of energy	Brooding, self-pity pessimism
Diminished ability to think or concentrate Indecisiveness	Lack of reactivity

Source: Endicott (1984).

depression (total = 13 per cent) were found utilizing *RDC* high-threshold criteria and high-threshold Endicott criteria.

Other depressive disorders

In addition to major depression, there are other *DSM-IV* diagnoses that commonly present in terminally ill patients that have depressed mood as a central presenting feature. Minor depression is similar to major depression, but requires fewer symptoms in order to qualify for a diagnosis (two to four symptoms in total). Dysthymia, in contrast, is defined as a chronic condition characterized by low-grade depressive symptoms that persist for at least two years. Adjustment disorder with depressed mood, on the other hand, describes a relatively short-lived maladaptive reaction to stress. This diagnosis requires that a patient's depressive response to the stressor must be 'in excess of a normal and expectable reaction'. If applied too loosely, the diagnosis of adjustment disorder can pathologize the experience of some patients by applying a psychiatric label on what may be a normal display of grief. Therefore, a comprehensive assessment of current and past depressive symptoms is essential in order to distinguish the above syndromes and subsequently determine appropriate treatment.

Risk factors for depression in the terminally ill

Gender

One of the most consistent results across epidemiological studies within the general population has been that women have rates of major depressive disorder that are approximately double those of men (Weissman *et al.* 1996). This finding leads to the hypothesis that women might also be more likely to become depressed in the face of life-threatening illness. In fact, some studies have indeed found higher levels of depressive symptoms and distress among women cancer patients (Stommel *et al.* 1993), including patients at an advanced terminal stage. Although gender is perceived to be a major risk for depression, it should be treated with caution among the terminally ill, as men may be more vulnerable to depression in this population.

Age

Epidemiological studies suggest that depressive disorders are more common among younger adults (that is, under age 45 years) than older adults. However, the expectation that this would translate into higher rates of depression among younger cancer patients must be tempered by the fact that cancer is a disease that predominantly affects older people. Nevertheless, a number of studies have identified the same trend and found that younger cancer patients do indeed show higher rates of diagnosed depressive disorders (Levine *et al.* 1978; Kathol *et al.* 1990*b*) or self-reported distress. Factors that can contribute to the higher prevalence of depression in younger patients may include the feeling that life has been cut short and ambitions have not been realized, concerns about the welfare of one's dependants, and also the methodological issue that younger people may be more willing to acknowledge psychological symptoms.

Prior history of depression

There is a growing recognition that for some individuals, depression can be a chronic or recurrent disorder. Within the general population, a prior episode of depression appears to be one of the stronger risk factors that predict the onset of new episodes. A number of studies have also found that patients with cancer who are currently depressed are more likely to report prior episodes from earlier periods in their lives (Hughes 1985). In this context, the struggle with life-threatening illness is clearly a major stressor that may precipitate an episode of depression in individuals who are particularly vulnerable (Harrison and Maguire 1994).

Social support

In studies of the general population, deficits in the adequacy of one's social support network have often been related to clinical depression (Bruce and Hoff 1994). The experience of social support is also thought to play a role in the psychological adjustment of patients with serious medical illness and has been found to be associated with depression in the terminally ill. The physical and psychosocial stressors associated with cancer are likely to result in a greater need for all forms of support. The provision of support may depend on family members, who are under considerable strain, as they attempt to cope with the life-threatening illness of a loved one. Furthermore, many patients with good relationships hesitate to add to their family's burden and avoid discussing their emotional state, which can intensify the sense of isolation. This cycle of isolating events can cause the patient to withdraw, and become depressed.

Functional status

Decreasing physical ability is correlated with measures of depression or distress (Kaasa *et al.* 1993; Williamson and Schulz 1995). Of course, functional ability is likely to decrease with the progression of the disease, so patients with more advanced illness appear to have the greatest risk for a number of psychiatric disorders. As patients receiving palliative care lose functional abilities, a sense of helplessness, dependency, deterioration, and confrontation with their own inevitable may fuel depressive symptomatology.

Pain

There is now a considerable body of evidence indicating that studies of patients with cancer have found an association between increased pain and reports of depression and such a link is indeed reliable across a range of settings and methods of assessment (Massie and Holland 1987; Chochinov *et al.* 1995; Glover *et al.* 1995). While the magnitude of the correlations are not especially high, the clinical implications are substantial. Recently, research has begun to shift from merely demonstrating that there is an association between pain and depression to considering more precisely what the nature of the causal link might be. Not only may uncontrolled pain increase depression, but also depression may result in an amplification of the pain experience (Spiegel and Bloom 1983).

Cancer and treatment-related factors

Specific types of cancers themselves, the subsequent disease process, as well as treatment related side-effects may induce depressive symptoms. Some sites of cancer are associated with depression beyond the level of the expected reactive symptoms. Tumours that originate in or metastasize to the central nervous system have the potential to cause depressive symptoms (Brown and Paraskevas 1982). Pancreatic cancer is also associated with depression (Shakin and Holland 1988) as are metabolic complications such as hypercalcaemia, most often associated with cancer of the breast and lung. These remote effects may be due to several factors, including toxins secreted by the tumour, autoimmune reactions, viral infections, nutritional deficits, and neuroendocrine dysfunction (McDaniel *et al.* 1995). Problems such as weight loss,

Table 6.6 Causes of depression in patients with advanced stage cancer

Uncontrolled pain

Metabolic abnormalities

Hypercalcemia, sodium or potassium imbalance, anemia, deficiencies in vitamins B_{12} or folate

Endocrinological abnormalities

Hyper- or hypothyroidism, adrenal insufficiency

Medications

Steroids, interferon and interleukin-2, methyldopa, reserpine, barbituates, propranolol, some antibiotics (amphotericin B), some chemotherapeutic agents (vincristine, vinblastine, procarbazine, L-asparaginase)

fatigue, sleep disturbance, and poor concentration are common symptoms of the disease process in cancer, and they can also be associated with the toxic side-effects of treatment. These treatments include corticosteroids (Stiefel *et al.* 1989), as well as various chemotherapy medications and radiotherapy protocols. More recently treatment with cytokine interferon alpha treatments have also been shown to induce symptoms of depression (Musselman *et al.* 2000). These risk factors are summarized in Table 6.6.

Existential concerns

In UK and US medical practice, it is very uncommon for patients with cancer not to be informed of their diagnosis. This has not always been the case, however; nor is it the case presently in some other societies. Reports from India (Alexander *et al.* 1993) and Poland (Walden-Galuszko 1996) show that patients who are unaware of the nature of their illness have substantially lower rates of psychiatric morbidity than do patients who have a more accurate appraisal of their circumstances. The recognition that one is facing a life-threatening crisis may bring with it a greater focus on existential concerns regarding unfulfilled ambitions, past regrets, meaning in life, and the maintenance of dignity and self-control, as well as social concerns about the welfare of one's family. In a study of sources of distress among patients with cancer, Noyes *et al.* (1990) found that items related to a loss of meaning showed higher correlation with scores on a depression inventory that did items pertaining to physical symptoms, medical treatment, or social isolation. The relationship of existential distress to depressive syndromes among patients who are terminally ill is worthy of further investigation in future research.

Suicide and the desire for hastened death in the terminally ill

Occasional thoughts of suicide are quite common in patients in palliative care settings and appear to act as a 'steam valve' for patients to cope with their feelings (Breitbart *et al.* 1993). However, persistent suicidal ideation is relatively infrequent and limited to patients in the context of psychiatric complications, such as depression. Patients with advanced cancer are at highest vulnerability because they are most likely to have such cancer complications such as pain, depression, delirium, and loss of autonomy, as well as strong feelings of helplessness and hopelessness. A review of the consultations done at the Memorial Sloan–Kettering Cancer Center demonstrated that 30 per cent of suicidal cancer patients had a major depression, 50 per cent were diagnosed with adjustment disorder at the time of evaluation, and about 20 per cent suffered from a delirium (Breitbart 1987).

Understanding why some patients with a terminal illness wish or seek to hasten their death remains an important element in both the physician-assisted suicide debate as well as the practice of palliative care. Although euthanasia and physician-assisted suicide have been distinguished legally and ethically from the administration of high-dose pain medication intended to relieve pain, there are still numerous questions to investigate such as understanding clearly the underlying wish and intent in expressing such demands as well as the factors associated with a patient's expression of a desire to die (Rosenfield *et al.* 2000). Despite the continued legal prohibitions against assisted suicide in most places, a substantial number of patients think about and discuss those alternatives with their physicians, family, and friends.

Desire for hastened death, the construct underlying requests for assisted suicide, euthanasia, and suicidal thoughts, remains an important element in the practice of palliative care. Recent research has focused on physical and psychological concerns, such as depression that may give rise to a desire for hastened death (Cassem 1987). Several studies have demonstrated that depression plays a significant role in the terminally ill patient's desire for hastened death. Breitbart *et al.* (2000) demonstrated in a sample of terminally ill cancer patients that both depression and hopelessness, characterized as a pessimistic cognitive style rather than an assessment of one's poor prognosis, appear to be independent determinants of desire for hastened death.

Assessment of suicide risk

Assessment of suicide risk and appropriate intervention are critical in palliative care settings. Furthermore, the myth that asking about suicidal thoughts put the 'idea into their head' is one that should be dispelled. In fact, patients often reconsider the idea of suicide when the legitimacy of these feelings and the patients need for a sense of control over death is acknowledged. A comprehensive evaluation, which includes a thorough history and inquiry into the patient's specific suicidal thoughts, plans, and intentions is required for any patient expressing interest in suicide or the related constructs of desire for hastened death and physician-assisted suicide (see Table 6.7). A clinician's ability to establish a report is essential, as they conduct a thorough evaluation on issues that include an assessment of risk, degree of intent, relevant history, quality of internal and external control, and the meaning behind the suicidal thoughts. In addition, mental status and adequacy of pain and symptom control should be determined.

Management of the suicidal patient

The response of a clinician to a patient's expression of desire for death, suicidal ideation, or request for assisted suicide has important and obvious implications on all

Table 6.7 Evaluation of suicidal patients in palliative care

Establish rapport using empathetic approach

Obtain patient's understanding of patient's illness and symptoms

Assess mental status

Assess vulnerability, pain control

Assess support system

Assess for history of alcohol/substance abuse

Inquire about recent losses/deaths

Obtain prior psychiatric history

Obtain family history

Obtain history of prior attempts or threats

Assess suicidal thinking, intent, and plans (see below)

Evaluate need for one-on-one observation in hospital or at home

Formulate treatment plan, short term and long term

Questions to assess for suicide
Open with a statement such as 'Most patients with cancer have passing thoughts about suicide, such as *"I might do something if things get bad enough ... "'*

Question	Rationale
Have you ever had thoughts like that?	Normalize
Any thoughts of not wanting to live or that it would be better if you were dead?	Ideation
Do you have any thoughts of suicide? Plans?	Intent
Have you thought about how you would do it?	Plan

Adapted from Breitbart (1990).

aspects of care, which impact on the patient, the patient's family, and staff. Once the setting has been made secure, these issues must be addressed both rapidly and thoughtfully, offering the patient a non-judgemental willingness to engage in a discussion of the factors that contribute to the suffering and despondency that leads patients to express such a desire for death. Most palliative care clinicians believe that effective management of physical and psychological symptoms will naturally prevent expressions of distress or requests for assisted suicide. Pharmacological interventions, including anti-depressants, analgesics, or narcoleptics should be utilized to treat symptoms of depression and any accompanying symptoms of anxiety, agitation, psychosis, or pain. The mobilization of the patients' support system may be highly effective as well. Furthermore, clinical interventions may need to be developed to more specifically address hopelessness and related constructs such as loss of meaning, demoralization, and spiritual distress that are especially prevalent near the end of life. Ultimately the palliative care clinician may not be able to prevent all suicides in all terminally ill patients. Prolonged suffering caused by poorly controlled symptoms can lead to such desperation, and it is the appropriate role of the palliative care team to provide effective management of physical and psychological symptoms as an alternative to desire for death, suicide, or request for assisted suicide.

Management of depression in palliative care

General principles

Once a depressive disorder has been identified in a terminally ill patient, the relationship with the primary medical caregiver or the mental health practitioner is the most important component of support for many patients with a serious illness. Optimally, these relationships are based on mutual trust, respect, and sensitivity. The ability to acknowledge the patient's distress, see the patient as a 'whole person', and respond to them on the basis of their own individual personal style and needs, tends to work best. Perhaps more than in any other clinical setting, maintaining ongoing contact with the depressed terminally ill patient is of critical importance. This not only ensures that patients will be continually re-evaluated, but also provides reassurance to patients that they will not be abandoned and that care will be forthcoming and available throughout their terminal course.

Psychosocial interventions

Depression in cancer patients is optimally managed utilizing a combination of supportive psychotherapy, cognitive–behavioural techniques, and anti-depressant medication (Maguire *et al.* 1985). For patients with cancer suffering from major depression, adjustment disorder, or dysthymia, there are a variety of psychosocial interventions with proven efficacy. These include individual psychotherapy, group psychotherapy, hypnotherapy, psycho-education, relaxation training and biofeedback, and self-help groups. Psychotherapy and cognitive–behavioural techniques are useful in the management of psychological distress in cancer patients and have been applied to the treatment of depressive and anxious symptoms related to cancer and cancer pain. Psychotherapeutic interventions, either in the form of individual or group counselling, have been shown to effectively reduce psychological distress and depressive symptoms in cancer patients (Spiegel and Wissler 1987). Cognitive–behavioural interventions, such as relaxation and distraction with pleasant imagery, have also been shown to decrease depressive symptoms in patients with mild to moderate levels of depression (Spiegel *et al.* 1981; Massie and Holland 1990). Due to the time-limited nature of treatment for the terminally ill however, supportive psychotherapy is a useful treatment approach to depression in the terminally ill patient. Finally, psychotherapy in conjunction with pharmacological treatment may be the quickest, most effective, and most comprehensive way to address patients' symptoms and distress near the end of life.

Pharmacological treatment of depression

Pharmacotherapy is the mainstay for treating terminally ill cancer patients meeting diagnosis criteria for major depression, as it often provides symptom reduction most quickly. Factors such as prognosis and the timeframe for treatment may play an important role in determining the type of pharmacotherapy for depression. A depressed patient with several months of life expectancy can afford to wait the two to four weeks it may take to respond to anti-depressants, such as selective serotonin re-uptake inhibitors (SSRIs). The depressed dying patient with less than three weeks to live may do best with a more rapidly acting psychostimulant. Patients who are within hours to days of death and are in distress are likely to benefit most from the use of sedation. These approaches will be discussed below.

There are a number of controlled studies of anti-depressant drug treatment for depressive disorders in cancer patients in general, but fewer that focus on the terminally ill. However, the efficacy of anti-depressants in the treatment of depression in cancer patients has been well established (Costa *et al.* 1985). Anti-depressants are only prescribed for the treatment of depression in one to three per cent of hospitalized cancer patients and only five per cent of terminally ill cancer patients. A survey of anti-depressant prescribing in the terminally ill found that out of 1046 cancer patients, only 10 per cent received anti-depressants, 76 per cent of whom did not receive them until the last two weeks of life (Lloyd-Williams *et al.* 1999). As discussed earlier, depressive symptoms are estimated to be present in a quarter of cancer patients. Therefore, it can be concluded that many depressed patients with advanced cancer never receive appropriate pharmacological treatment or receive it only in the final two weeks of life, when it is too late for a treatment response. Table 6.8 outlines the anti-depressant medications used in advanced cancer patients.

Selective serotonin re-uptake inhibitors

Selective serotonin re-uptake inhibitors are commonly the first line of treatment in advanced cancer patients with an estimated lifespan of a few weeks or longer, because of their safety and low side-effect profile. It is good practice 'to start low and go slow'

Table 6.8 Anti-depressant medications used in palliative care settings

Drug	Therapeutic daily dosage (mg) orally
Psychostimulants	
Dextroamphetamine	5–30
Methylphenidate	5–30
Modafinil	50–400
Pemoline	37.5–150
Second generation anti-depressants	
Serotonin selective re-uptake inhibitors	
Fluoxetine	10–40
Paroxetine	10–40
Citalopram	20–40
Fluvoxamine	50–300
Sertraline	50–200

Table 6.8 continued

Drug	Therapeutic daily dosage (mg) orally
Serotonin/ norepinephrine reuptake inhibitor	
Venlafaxine	37.5–225
5-HT$_2$ antagonists/ serotonin/ norepinephrine re-uptake inhibitors	
Nefazodone	100–500
Trazodone	150–300
Norepinephrine/dopamine re-uptake inhibitor	
Buproprion	200–450
alpha-2 antagonist/5-HT$_2$ antagonist	
Mirtazepine	7.5–30
Tricyclic anti-depressants	
Secondary amine	
Desipramine	25–125
Nortriptyline	25–125
Tertiary amine	
Amitriptyline	25–125
Doxepin	25–125
Imipramine	25–125
Clomipramine	25–125
Heterocyclic anti-depressants	
Maprotiline	50–75
Amoxapine	100–150
Monoamine oxidase inhibitors	
Isocarboxazid	20–40
Phenelzine	30–60
Tranylcypromine	20–40
Mood stabilizers	
Lithium carbonate	600–1200
Benzodiazepines	
Alprazolam	0.75–6.00

Adapted from Massie and Holland (1990).

in cancer patients in order to reduce gastrointestinal side-effects of nausea and transient weight loss. The SSRIs are safe with chemotherapeutic agents but should be avoided in patients receiving procarbazine for management of some haematological malignancies because procarbazine is a monoamine oxidase inhibitor (MAOI).

The SSRIs have a number of features that are advantageous for cancer patients. They have a very low affinity for adrenergic, cholinergic, and histamine receptors, thus accounting for negligible orthostatic hypotension, urinary retention, memory impairment, sedation, or reduced awareness. They do not therefore require therapeutic drug-level monitoring, have not been found to cause clinically significant alterations in cardiac conduction, and are generally favourably tolerated along with a wider margin of safety than the tricyclic anti-depressants (TCAs) in the event of an overdose.

Most of the side-effects of SSRIs result from their selective central and peripheral serotonin re-uptake properties. These include increased intestinal motility (for example, loose stools, nausea, and vomiting) insomnia, headaches, and sexual dysfunction. Some patients may experience anxiety, tremor, restlessness, and akathisia (the latter is relatively rare but it can be problematic for the terminally ill patient with Parkinson's disease). These side-effects tend to be dose related and may be problematic for patients with advanced disease. Initially adding a benzodiazepine with the SSRI helps to prevent the common side-effects of anxiety, restlessness, and akasthisia.

There are five SSRIs available on the market including sertraline, fluoxetine, paroxetine, citalopram, and fluvoxamine. With the exception of fluoxetine, whose elimination half-life is two to four days, the SSRIs have an elimination half-life of about 24 hours. Fluoxetine is the only SSRI with a potent active metabolite—norfluoxetine—whose elimination half-life is 7–14 days. Fluoxetine can cause mild nausea and a brief period of increased anxiety as well as appetite suppression that usually lasts for a period of several weeks. Some patients can experience transient weight loss but weight usually returns to baseline level. This has not been a limiting factor in the use of fluoxetine in cancer patients. Fluoxetine and norfluoxetine do not reach a steady state for five to six weeks, compared with 4–14 days for paroxetine, fluvoxamine, and sertraline. These differences are important, especially for the terminally ill patient in whom a switch from an SSRI to another anti-depressant is being considered. If a switch to a monamine oxidase inhibitor is required, the washout period for fluoxetine will be at least five weeks, given the potential drug interactions between these two agents. Until it has been studied further in cancer, fluoxetine should be used cautiously in the debilitated dying patient. Paroxetine, fluvoxamine, and sertraline, on the other hand, require considerably shorter washout periods (10–14 days) under similar circumstances.

All the SSRIs have the ability to inhibit the hepatic isoenzyme P450 11D6, with sertraline and fluvoxamine being least potent in this regard. Since SSRIs are dependent upon hepatic metabolism, this becomes significant with respect to dose–plasma level ratios and drug interactions. For the elderly patient with advanced disease, the dose–response curve for sertraline appears to be relatively linear, whereas for the others, particularly for paroxetine, small dosage increases can result in dramatic elevations in plasma levels. Paroxetine and fluoxetine inhibit the hepatic enzymes responsible for their own clearance (Preskorn 1993). The co-administration of these medications with other drugs that are dependent on this enzyme system for their catabolism (for example, tricyclics, phenothiazines, and quinidine) should be done cautiously. Fluvoxamine has been shown in some instances to elevate the blood levels of propranolol and warfarin by as much as two-fold and should thus not be prescribed together with these agents.

For advanced cancer patients, SSRIs can be started at approximately half the usual starting dose used in a healthy patient. Titration of fluoxetine can begin on 5 mg (available in liquid form) given once daily (preferably in the morning) with a range of 10–40 mg per day; given its long half-life, some patients may only require this drug every second day. Paroxetine can be started at 10 mg once daily (either morning or evening) and has a therapeutic range of 10–40 per day. Fluvoxamine, which tends to be somewhat more sedating, can be started at 25 mg (in the evenings) and has a therapeutic range of 50–300 mg. Sertraline can be initiated at 50 mg (morning or evening) and titrated within a range of 50–200 mg per day. Citalopram can be initiated at 10 mg (in the morning) and titrated within a range of 10–40 mg per day. If patients experience activating effects of SSRIs, they should not be given at bedtime but rather moved earlier into the day. Ensuring the patient is not taking the medication on an empty stomach can reduce gastrointestinal upset.

Serotonin–norepinephrine re-uptake inhibitor

Venlafaxine (Effexor) is the only anti-depressant in this class. It is a potent inhibitor of neuronal serotonin and norepinephrine re-uptake and appears to have no significant affinity for muscarinic, histamine, or alpha$_1$-adrenergic receptors. Some patients may experience an increase in blood pressure, especially at doses above the recommended initiating dose. Compared with all other available anti-depressants, its protein binding (<35 per cent) is very low. Few protein binding-induced drug interactions are thus expected. Venlafaxine should not be used in patients receiving monamine oxidase inhibitors. Its side-effect profile tends to generally be well tolerated with few discontinuations. While there are currently no data addressing its use in the depressed cancer patient, its pharmacokinetic properties and side-effect profile suggest it may have a role to play.

Nefazodone

Nefazodone and trazodone are chemically related anti-depressants that block post-synaptic 5-HT$_2$ receptors. Nefazodone is much less sedating than trazodone but more likely to cause gastrointestinal activation. Nefazodone can be started at 50 mg at bedtime and titrated within a range of 100–500 mg per day. Nefazodone does not have any sexual dysfunction side-effect.

Trazodone

If given in sufficient doses (100–300 mg per day), trazodone can be an effective anti-depressant. In addition to its blockade of post-synaptic 5-HT$_2$ receptors, it also has considerable affinity for alpha$_1$-adrenoceptors and may thus predispose patients to orthostatic hypotension and its problematic sequelae, that is, falls. Trazodone is very sedating and in low doses (100 mg) is helpful in the treatment of the depressed cancer patient with insomnia. Weight gain is an additional common and useful side-effect in patients with anorexia. Both nefazodone and trazodone can be used alone or in combination with SSRIs. Lack of anti-cholinergic side-effects with these medications is helpful in treating patients prone to delirium and cognitive dysfunction.

Mirtazapine

Mirtazapine is the 6-aza analogue of the tetracyclic anti-depressant mianserin. Mirtazapine enhances central noradrenergic and serotonergic activity with blockade of central presynaptic alpha$_2$ inhibitory receptors and postsynaptic serotonin 5-HT$_2$ and 5-HT$_3$ receptors. It compares favourably with amitriptyline and trazodone, with further studies needed to compare the clinical efficacy of mirtazapine to serotonin re-uptake inhibitors. Mirtazapine improves appetite resulting in weight gain, which is desirable in cancer patients. In addition, the marked sedative effect of this medication proves quite useful in patients with sleeping difficulties.

Tricyclic anti-depressants

The application of TCAs specifically to cancer patients requires a careful risk–benefit ratio analysis, especially when used in patients with advanced cancer. Although nearly 70 per cent of patients treated with a tricyclic for non-psychotic depression can anticipate a positive response, their side-effect profile can be troublesome for cancer patients. Constipation and dry mouth are undesirable in cancer patients, especially those on opioids, and response time is also long. Their multiple pharmacodynamic actions accounting for these side-effects include blockade of muscarinic cholinergic receptors, alpha-adrenoceptors, and H$_1$-histamine receptors. The tertiary amines (amitriptyline, doxepin, and imipramine) have a greater propensity to cause side-effects than do secondary amines (nortriptyline and desipramine). The anti-cholinergic actions of TCAs can also cause serious tachycardia. Their quinidine-like effects can lead to arrhythmias by delaying the conduction through the His–Purkinje system.

Tricyclic anti-depressants should be started at low doses (10–25 mg) and increased in 10–25 mg increments every two to four days until a therapeutic dose is attained or side-effects become a dose-limiting factor. Depressed cancer patients often achieve a therapeutic response at significantly lower doses of TCAs (25–125 mg) than are necessary in the physically well (150–300 g). The choice of which specific TCA to use depends on a variety of factors including the nature of the underlying medical condition, the characteristics of the depressive episode, past responses to anti-depressant therapy, and the specific drug side-effect profile. For depressed cancer patients, the choice of TCA is made on the basis of a side-effect profile that will be least incompatible with the patient's overall medical condition. Most tricyclics are available as rectal suppositories for patients who are no longer able to take medication orally. Most importantly, therapeutic response to TCAs, as with all anti-depressants, has a latency time of three to six weeks.

Monamine oxidase inhibitors

In general, MAOIs are rarely used in cancer settings, including palliative care facilities. Patients who receive MAOIs must avoid foods rich in tyramine, sympathomimetic drugs (amphetamines and methylphenidate), and medications containing phenyl-propanolamine and pseudoephedrine (Breitbart and Mermelstein 1992). The combination of these agents with MAOIs may cause hypertensive crisis, leading to strokes and fatalities. MAOIs in combination with opioid analgesics have also been reported to be associated with myoclonus and delirium and must therefore be used together cautiously (Breitbart 1988). MAOIs can also cause considerable orthostatic hypotension.

The new reversible inhibitors of monoamine oxidase-A (RIMAs) may reduce some of the problems associated with the older MAOIs. There are no studies on the role of RIMAs in the depressed cancer patient but there are interesting theoretical reasons to suggest that they may eventually have a larger role to play than the non-selective MAOIs. Moclobemide, a RIMA recently introduced onto the Canadian market, appears to be loosely bound to the MAO-A receptor and is thus relatively easily displaced by tyramine from its binding sight. It has a very short half-life, which further reduces the possibility of any prolonged adverse effects, for example, hypertensive crisis. Dietary restrictions for avoiding tyramine-containing foods are thus not required. The side-effect profile of moclobemide is far more favourable than for non-selective MAOIs and tends to be well tolerated. Although the risk of hypertensive crisis is significantly reduced, it is not however entirely eliminated and MAOIs are likely to remain second-line anti-depressants.

Psychostimulants

Psychostimulants currently approved for use in cancer patients include methylphenidate, dextroamphetamine, pemoline, and modafinil and all have a rapid onset of action. They have been shown to be rapidly effective anti-depressants especially in the cancer setting (Breitbart and Mermelstein 1992; Bruera et al. 1986; Fernandez et al. 1987; Olin and Masand 1996; Burns and Eisendrath 1994). Several investigators have demonstrated the efficacy of methylphenidate in the treatment of depression in advanced cancer patients, reporting rapid onset of action (one to three days) and response rates as high as 85 per cent. The chewable form of pemoline is especially favourable in those who can no longer tolerate the oral route but can utilize buccal absorption.

In relatively low doses, psychostimulants stimulate appetite, promote a sense of well-being, and improve feelings of weakness and fatigue in cancer patients. Treatment with dextroamphetamine or methylphenidate usually begins with a dose of 2.5 mg at 8:00 AM and at noon. The dosage is slowly increased over several days until a desired effect is achieved or side-effects (overstimulation, anxiety, insomnia, paranoia, and confusion) intervene. Patients are usually maintained on methylphenidate for one to two months and approximately two-thirds will be able to be withdrawn from methylphenidate without a recurrence of depressive symptoms. Tolerance will develop and adjustment of dose may be necessary. An additional benefit of stimulants is that they have been shown to reduce sedation secondary to opioid analgesics and provide adjuvant analgesics in cancer patients (Bruera et al. 1987). Common side-effects of stimulants include nervousness, overstimulation, mild increase in blood pressure and pulse rate, and tremor. More rare side-effects include dyskinesias or motor tics as well as paranoid psychosis or exacerbation of an underlying and unrecognized confusional state.

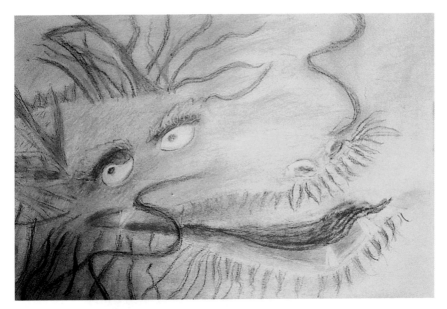

Plate 1 *So afraid* (see p. 4).

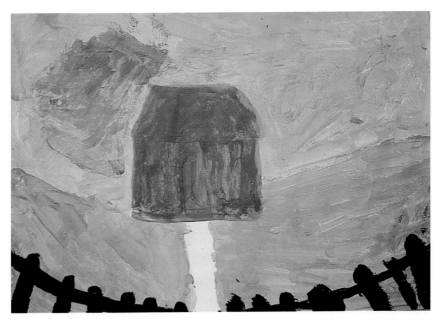

Plate 2 *The threat of losing home* (see p. 35).

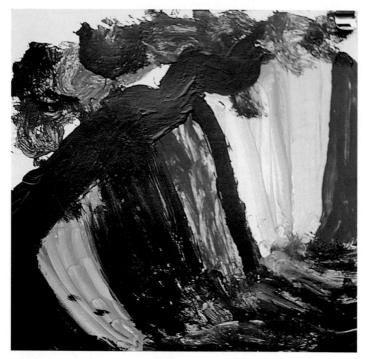

Plate 3 *A hole so deep* (see p. 81). (see p. 81)

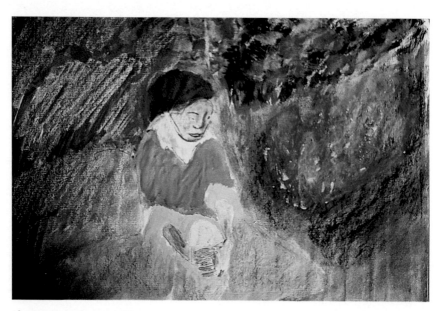

Plate 4 *Alone* (see p. 149). (see p. 149)

Recently, modafinil, a new and novel psychostimulant, was approved for use in the USA. Although more controlled studies need to be completed, early case series reports suggest its efficacy as an anti-depressant. Modafinil is a novel psychostimulant that has sympathomimetic properties but does not have a similar pharmacological profile to the other sympathomimetic amines. A case series by Menza *et al.* (2000) showed modafinil to be a useful augmenting agent in treatment-resistant depression, particularly when patients complain of fatigue as one of their symptoms. In this series, modafinil was used in combination with a number of different anti-depressants and anti-convulsants, including SSRIs and venlafaxine. The addition of modafinil was well tolerated and led to a marked reduction in depressive symptoms in all seven patients. Modafinil should be given in the morning and can be started at a dose of 100 mg for most patients. Starting at 50 mg is advisable for elderly or frail patients. The dose can then be titrated upwards.

Pemoline

Pemoline is another psychostimulant that is chemically unrelated to amphetamine. There are several advantages for using pemoline in cancer patients. A unique property of pemoline is its availability in chewable tablet form with good absorption through the buccal mucosa, which is very useful in cancer patients who have difficulty swallowing or intestinal obstruction. Pemoline is as effective as methylphenidate and dextroamphetamine in the treatment of depression in cancer patients (Bruera *et al.* 1986). Pemoline can be started at a dose of 18.75 mg in the morning and at noon and increased gradually over days. Typically patients require 75 mg a day or less. Pemoline should be used with caution in patients with liver impairment and liver function tests should be monitored periodically with longer-term treatment (Nehra *et al.* 1990).

Lithium carbonate

Patients receiving lithium prior to their cancer diagnosis should be maintained on the drug throughout their treatment although close monitoring will be necessary. Maintenance doses of lithium may need reduction in seriously ill patients. Lithium should be prescribed with caution for patients receiving *cis*-platinum because of the potential nephrotoxicity of both drugs (Greenberg *et al.* 1993).

Electroconvulsive therapy

Occasionally, it is necessary to consider electroconvulsive therapy (ECT) for depressed cancer patients who have depression with psychotic features or in whom treatment with anti-depressants poses unacceptable side-effects. Although generally a safe treatment for medically ill patients, the use of ECT is often impractical in a palliative care setting and therefore rarely utilized.

Conclusions

Depression is a common complication among patients receiving end-of-life care, which continues to be under-recognized and remains a source of considerable suffering. The underdiagnosis and undertreatment of depression has a substantial impact on the quality of the last weeks of life for the terminally ill patient. Awareness of the risk factors associated with the development of depression, as well as the utilization of methods of accurate assessment of depression, can increase the likelihood of identifying these patients. Both pharmacological and non-pharmacological treatments for depression are often highly effective in patients with advanced cancer and should be readily utilized. The amelioration of depression is essential in order to provide effective and comprehensive palliative care, as it will minimize prolonged suffering, maximize the potential for a meaningful existence, and help provide greater quality of life near the end of life.

References

Alexander PJ, Dinesh N, Vidyasagar MS (1993). Psychiatric morbidity among cancer patients and its relationship with awareness of illness and expectations about treatment outcome. *Acta Oncol* **32**:623–6.

American Psychiatric Association (1994). *Diagnostic and statistical manual of mental disorders.* 4th edn. Washington, DC: American Psychiatric Association.

Breitbart W (1987). Suicide in cancer patients. *Oncology* **1**:49–53.

Breitbart WS (1988). Psychiatric complications of cancer. In: Brain MC (ed.). *Current therapy in hematology oncology, Vol. 3.* Toronto and Philadelphia: Decker. pp. 268–74.

Breitbart W. (1990). Cancer pain and suicide. In: Foley K, Bonica JJ, Ventafridda V (ed.). *Advances in pain research and therapy, Vol. 16.* New York: Raven Press. p. 409.

Breitbart W, Mermelstein H (1992). Pemoline. An alternative psychostimulant for the management of depressive disorders in cancer patients. *Psychosomatics* **33**:352–6.

Breitbart W, Levenson JA, Passik SD (1993). Terminally ill cancer patients. In: Breitbart W, Holland JC (ed.). *Psychiatric aspects of symptom management in cancer patients.* Washington, DC: American Psychiatric Press. pp. 192–94.

Breitbart W, Bruera E, Chochinov H, Lynch M (1995). Neuropsychiatric syndromes and psychological symptoms in patients with advanced cancer. *J Pain Sympt Management* **10**:131–41.

Breitbart W, Chochinov HM, Passik S (1998). Psychiatric aspects of palliative care. In: Doyle D, Hanks GEC, McDonald N (ed.). *Oxford textbook of palliative medicine.* New York: Oxford University Press. pp. 933–54.

Breitbart W, Rosenfeld B, Pessin H, Kavim M, Funesti-Esten J, Galietta M *et al.* (2000). Depression, hopelessness, and desire for hastened death in terminally ill patients with cancer. *JAMA* **284**:2907–11.

Brown JH, Paraskevas F (1982). Cancer and depression: cancer presenting with depressive illness: an autoimmune disease? *Br J Psychiat* **141**:227–32.

Bruce ML, Hoff RA (1994). Social and physical health risk factors for first-onset major depressive disorder in a community sample. *Soc Psychiat Psychiatr Epidemiol* **29**:165–71.

Bruera E, Carraro S, Roca E, Barugel M, Chacon R (1986). Double-blind evaluation of the effects of mazindol on pain, depression, anxiety, appetite, and activity in terminal cancer patients. *Cancer Treat Rep* **70**:295–8.

Bruera E, Chadwick S, Brenneis C, Hanson J, MacDonald RN (1987). Methylphenidate associated with narcotics for the treatment of cancer pain. *Cancer Treat Rep* **71**:67–70.

Bukberg J, Penman D, Holland JC (1984). Depression in hospitalized cancer patients. *Psychom Med* **46**(3):199–212.

Burns MM, Eisendrath SJ (1994). Dextroamphetamine treatment for depression in terminally ill patients. *Psychosomatics* **35**:80–3.

Cassem NH (1987). The dying patient. In: Hackett TP, Cassem, NH (ed.). *Massachusetts general hospital handbook of general hospital psychiatry*. Littleton, Massachusetts: PSG Publishing. pp. 332–52.

Chochinov HM, Wilson KG, Enns M, Lander S (1994). Prevalence of depression in the terminally ill: effects of diagnostic criteria and symptom threshold judgments. *Am J Psychiat* **15**:537–40.

Chochinov HM, Wilson KG, Enns M *et al.* (1995): Desire for death in the terminally ill. *Am J Psychiat* **152**:1185–91.

Costa D, Mogos I, Toma T (1985). Efficacy and safety of mianserin in the treatment of depression of women with cancer. *Acta Psychiatr Scand* (**suppl 320**):85–92.

Derogatis LR, Morrow GR, Fetting J, Penman D, Piasetsky S, Schmale A *et al.* (1983). The prevalence of psychiatric disorders among cancer patients. *JAMA* **249**:751–7.

Endicott J. (1984). Measurement of depression in patients with cancer. *Cancer* **53**:2243–8.

Endicott J, Spitzer RL (1978). A diagnostic interview: the schedule for affective disorders and schizophrenia. *Arch Gen Psychiat* **35**:837–44.

Evans DL, McCartney CF, Nemeroff CB *et al.* (1986). Depression in women treated for gynecological cancer: clinical and neuroendocrine assessment. *Am J Psychiatry* **143**(4):447–52.

Fernandez F, Adams F, Holmes VF, Levy JK, Neidhart M (1987). Methylphenidate for depressive disorders in cancer patients. An alternative to standard antidepressants. *Psychosomatics* **28**:455–61.

Glover J, Dibble SL, Dodd MJ, Miaskowski C (1995). Mood states of oncology outpatients: does pain make a difference? *J Pain Sympt Management* **10**:120–8.

Greenberg DB, Younger J, Kaufman SD (1993). Management of lithium in patients with cancer. *Psychosomatics* **34**:388–94.

Harrison J, Maguire P (1994). Predictors of psychiatric morbidity in cancer patients [see comments]. *Br J Psychiat* **165**:593–8.

Hughes JE (1985). Depressive illness and lung cancer. I. Depression before diagnosis. *Eur J Surg Oncol* **11**:15–20.

Kaasa S, Malt U, Hagen S, Wist E, Moum T, Kvikstad A (1993). Psychological distress in cancer patients with advanced disease. *Radiother Oncol* **27**:193–7.

Kathol RG, Mutgi A, Williams J, Clamon G, Noyes R Jr (1990a). Diagnosis of major depression in cancer patients according to four sets of criteria. *Am J Psychiat* **147**:1021–4.

Kathol RG, Noyes R Jr, Williams J, Mutgi A, Carroll B, Perry P (1990b). Diagnosing depression in patients with medical illness. *Psychosomatics* **31**:434–40.

Kelsen DP, Portenoy RK, Thaler HT *et al.* (1995). Pain and depression in patients with newly diagnosed pancreas cancer. *J Clin Oncol* **13**(3):748–55.

Lansky SB, List MA, Hermann CA *et al.* (1985). Absence of major depressive disorders in female cancer patients. *J Clin Oncol* **3**(11):1553–60.

Levine PM, Silberfarb PM, Lipowski ZJ (1978). Mental disorders in cancer patients: a study of 100 psychiatric referrals. *Cancer* **42**:1385–91.

Lloyd-Williams M, Friedman T, Rudd N (1999). A survey of antidepressant prescribing in the terminally ill. *Palliative Med* **13**:243–8.

Lynn J, Teno JM, Phillips RS, Wu A, Desbiens N, Harrold J et al. (1997). Perceptions by family members of the dying experience of older and seriously ill patients. SUPPORT Investigators. Study to Understand Prognoses and Preferences for Outcomes and Risks of Treatments [see comments]. *Ann Intern Med* **126**:97–106.

Maguire P, Hopwood P, Tarrier N, Howell T (1985). Treatment of depression in cancer patients. *Acta Psychiatr Scand* (**suppl 320**):81–4.

Massie MJ (1989). Depression. In: Holland JC, Rowland JH (ed.). *Handbook of Psychooncology: psychological care of the patient with cancer.* New York: Oxford University Press. pp. 283–90.

Massie MJ, Holland JC (1987). The cancer patient with pain: psychiatric complications and their management. *Med Clin N Am* **71**:243–58.

Massie MJ, Holland JC (1990). Depression and the cancer patient. *J Clin Psychiatry* **51** (**suppl**):12–17 (and discussion 18–19).

McDaniel JS, Musselman DL, Porter MR, Reed DA, Nemeroff CB (1995). Depression in patients with cancer. Diagnosis, biology, and treatment. *Arch Gen Psychiat* **52**:89–99.

Menza MA, Kaufman KR, Castellanos AM (2000). Modafinil augmentation of antidepressant treatment in depression. *J Clin Psychiat* **61**:378–81.

Minagawa H, Uchitomi Y, Yamawaki S, Ishitani K (1996). Psychiatric morbidity in terminally ill cancer patients. A prospective study [see comments]. *Cancer* **78**:1131–7.

Musselman DL, Lawson DH, Gumnick JF (2000). Paroxetine for the prevention of depression induced by high dose interferon alfa. *N Engl J Med* **344**:961–6.

Nehra A, Mullick F, Ishak KG, Zimmerman HJ (1990). Pemoline-associated hepatic injury. *Gastroenterology* **99**:1517–9.

Noyes R Jr, Kathol RG, Debelius-Enemark P, Williams J, Mutgi A, Snelzer M et al. (1990). Distress associated with cancer as measured by the illness distress scale. *Psychosomatics* **31**:321–30.

Olin J, Masand P (1996). Psychostimulants for depression in hospitalized cancer patients. *Psychosomatics* **37**:57–62.

Preskorn SH (1993). Recent pharmacologic advances in antidepressant therapy for the elderly. *Am J Med* **94**:2S–12S.

Razavi D, Delvaux N, Farvacques C, Robaye E (1990). Screening for adjustment disorders and major depressive disorders in cancer in-patients [see comments]. *Br J Psychiatry* **156**:79–83.

Robins LN, Helzer JE, Croughan J, Ratcliff KS (1981). National Institute of Mental Health Diagnostic Interview Schedule. Its history, characteristics, and validity. *Arch Gen Psychiat* **38**:381–9.

Rosenfeld B, Krivo S, Breitbart W, Chochinov HM (2000). Suicide, assisted suicide, and euthanasia in the terminally ill. In: Chochinov HM, Breitbart W (ed.). *Handbook of psychiatry in palliative medicine.* New York: Oxford University Press. pp. 51–62.

Shakin EJ, Holland J (1988). Depression and pancreatic cancer *J Pain Sympt Management* **3**:194–8.

Spiegel D, Bloom JR (1983). Pain in metastatic breast cancer. *Cancer* **52**:341–5.

Spiegel D, Wissler T (1987). Using family consultation as psychiatric aftercare for schizophrenic patients. *Hosp Community Psychiat* **38**:1096–9.

Spiegel D, Bloom JR, Yalom I (1981). Group support for patients with metastatic cancer. A randomized outcome study. *Arch Gen Psychiat* **38**:527–33.

Spitzer RL, Endicott J, Robins E (1978). Research diagnostic criteria: rationale and reliability. *Arch Gen Psychiat* **35**:773–82.

Spitzer RL, Williams JBW, Gibbon M, First MB (1990). *Structured clinical interview for DSM-III-R.* Washington, DC: American Psychiatric Press.

Spitzer RL, Williams JB, Kroenke K *et al.* (1994). Utility of a new procedure for diagnosing mental disorders in primary care. The PRIME-MD 1000 study [see comments]. *JAMA* **272**:1749–56.

Stiefel FC, Breitbart WS, Holland JC (1989). Corticosteroids in cancer: neuropsychiatric complications. *Cancer Invest* **7**:479–91.

Stommel M, Given BA, Given CW, Kalaian HA, Schulz R, McCorkle R (1993). Gender bias in the measurement properties of the Center for Epidemiologic Studies Depression Scale (CES-D). *Psychiat Res* **49**:239–50.

Walden-Galuszko Kd (1996). Prevalence of psychological morbidity in terminally ill cancer patients. *Psycho-oncology* **5**:45–9.

Weissman MM, Bland RC, Canino GJ *et al.* (1996). Cross-national epidemiology of major depression and bipolar disorder. *JAMA* **276**:293–9.

Williamson GM, Schulz R (1995). Activity restriction mediates the association between pain and depressed affect: a study of younger and older adult cancer patients. *Psychol Aging* **10**:369–78.

Chapter 7

Screening for depression in palliative care

Mari Lloyd-Williams

Introduction

'It's not only the pain in my leg, it's the pain in my heart and the pain in my mind.' David was twenty-one years old and dying of osteosarcoma—he was increasingly withdrawn, had an air of hopelessness and despair that did not resolve, and he died three weeks after we had the above conversation. In retrospect David was undoubtedly depressed, but as in so many cases of patients with advanced malignant disease, the depression was not diagnosed and therefore not treated until too late in the course of the illness for any therapeutic intervention to be beneficial. It can be so difficult to distinguish between what may be called 'appropriate' sadness at the end of life and a treatable depressive illness.

How much of a problem is depression at the end of life?

It is recognized that psychiatric disorders occur more frequently in cancer patients than in the general population (Breitbart et al. 1995; Block 2000). It is estimated that 50 per cent of patients will have no significant psychiatric symptoms, 30 per cent will have what is defined as an adjustment reaction and 20 per cent will have a formal psychiatric diagnosis, the most common being depression. It is estimated that for a quarter of all patients admitted to a palliative care unit, depression will be a significant symptom (Barraclough 1994). The prevalence of depression in the general population is 6–10 per cent, therefore a number of patients with advanced cancer may have a pre-existing psychiatric disorder and the advancing cancer will place these patients at greater risk of developing further episodes (Bergevin and Bergevin 1995). According to some studies, up to 80 per cent of the psychological and psychiatric morbidity that develops in cancer patients goes unrecognized and untreated (Maguire 1985). This low rate of detection is thought to be due to non-disclosure by patients who may feel either that they are wasting the doctor's time or that they are in some way to blame for their distress and therefore choose to hide it (Maguire and Howell 1995). Another factor may be the lack of confidence in diagnosing this symptom of many medical and nursing staff (Brugha 1993).

Hinton, a psychiatrist, carried out some of the earliest research work looking at the physical and mental distress of dying patients in 1963 (Hinton 1963). He studied 102 patients who were dying and compared them to hospital in-patients. He found that terminally ill patients had higher levels of both physical and emotional distress and that 24 per cent had depression. He concluded that depression had a significant association with the degree and duration of the terminal illness with patients under fifty years of age having greater physical and mental distress. Later work by Addington Hall and McCarthy (1995) looked at the caregivers' perception of symptoms in the last year and week of life. Perceptions of feeling low and miserable were reported by 69 per cent during the last year and 52 per cent during the last week of life. It must be stressed that these are caregivers' perceptions, which other research has shown tend to reflect the respondent rather than the patient's level of distress. Fulton (1997) found that 50 per cent of patients with breast cancer had symptoms of depression in the last few weeks of life. In Hughes' prospective study of 50 patients with advanced inoperable lung cancer (Hughes 1985), 16 per cent had a major depressive illness. Ramsay (1992) in a study of all referrals to a liaison psychiatry service during one year found that of the 26 patients were referred (10 per cent of the total number of patients admitted to the unit during the year), 50 per cent had a diagnosis of depression. All the above evidence suggests that depression is a real and distressing symptom for many patients in the last months and weeks of life.

Nursing staff have an important role in identifying patients who may have psychiatric symptoms (Valentine and Saunders 1989; McVey 1998). Nurses spend more time in direct patient contact enabling them to observe behaviour more closely and the nature of intimate nursing tasks may give an opportunity for patients to express any psychological distress. In a study of 100 oncology nurses caring for 475 patients on one particular day, Pasacreta and Massie (1990) used a questionnaire developed to help nurses identify patients with psychiatric symptoms. These nurses perceived that 55 per cent of patients had symptoms requiring further psychiatric evaluation—a higher figure than would be expected; the 55 per cent included 13 per cent already under psychiatric care. They concluded that although nurses may not be able to identify specific psychiatric disorders, they are skilful in recognizing significant psychological distress. All members of a multi-disciplinary team have a role to play in the diagnosis and management of depression.

How is depression diagnosed?

There are no universally accepted criteria for diagnosing depression in the terminally ill patient. In the physically healthy population, depression is diagnosed if patients have a persistent low mood and a least four of the following symptoms which are present most of the day and have been for the preceding two weeks:

(1) diminished interest or pleasure in all or almost all activities;

(2) Psychomotor retardation or agitation;

(3) feelings of worthlessness or excessive and inappropriate guilt;

(4) diminished ability to concentrate and think;

(5) recurrent thoughts of death and suicide;

(6) fatigue and loss of energy;

(7) significant weight loss or gain;

(8) insomnia or hypersomnia.

In patients with advanced cancer, symptoms 6–8 are almost universal and there has been considerable controversy as to whether physical symptoms should be included and, if included, their importance in diagnosing depression in the terminally ill. Casey (1994) suggested that symptoms such as feelings of worthlessness, helplessness, and hopelessness, feelings of excessive and inappropriate guilt, and thoughts of self-harm were particularly discriminating in those patients with advanced terminal cancer. Buckberg *et al.* (1984) believed that anorexia, weight loss, and low energy were such common symptoms in the medically ill that they proposed eliminating these somatic symptoms as criteria for diagnosis of depression. They also found that the point prevalence of major depression dropped from 42 to 24 per cent when all somatic symptoms were eliminated as criteria. The complex problem of deciding which symptoms may be attributable to the cancer and which may be due to depression has been discussed by Endicott (1984) who proposed that the somatic symptoms listed should be substituted in the patient with cancer, that is

(1) diminished concentration or slowed thinking; substituted by cannot be cheered up, does not smile, no response to good news or funny situations;

(2) poor appetite/weight gain, substituted by fearfulness or depressed appearance in body or face;

(3) insomnia/hypersomnia, substituted by social withdrawal or decreased talkativeness;

(4) loss of energy/fatigue, substituted by brooding, self pity, pessimism.

Endicott also stressed the importance of asking patients with cancer about suicidal ideation. Chochinov *et al.* (1994) compared the research diagnostic criteria with Endicott's revised criteria in 130 patients and suggested that small differences between investigators in the application of symptom severity thresholds can cause large differences in prevalence rates for depression. They also concluded that the inclusion of somatic symptoms only inflates the rates of diagnosis when these symptoms are used in conjunction with what he describes as a 'low threshold approach'. Cavanaugh (1984) reviewed the diagnosis of depression in the chronically medically ill and concluded that affective and cognitive symptoms are most useful and somatic symptoms, although less useful, could be used to support the diagnosis if they were severe and proportionate to the medical illness. Thus the debate on the use of somatic-type symptoms and diagnostic criteria still continues. A useful concept when considering whether a patient is depressed is that the patient who blames the illness for how they are feeling is probably experiencing sadness at their illness and condition whereas a patient who blames themselves for their illness and for how they are feeling, may well be depressed.

Strategies have been proposed for the management of depression in patients with advanced cancer (Haig 1992):

(1) good rapport should be established;

(2) thorough psychiatric assessment and relief of poorly controlled symptoms;

(3) underlying organic factors detected and treated where possible;

(4) normal sadness and grief at the end of life differentiated from those indicating a depressive disorder;

(5) supportive psychotherapy for the patients to reduce sense of isolation;

(6) family intervention to support relatives;

(7) use of selected anti-depressants.

Although these guidelines may be helpful, they do not detail what a thorough psychiatric assessment entails. Psychiatrists write the majority of papers discussing the psychiatric needs of terminally ill patients but it is not known how many patients receiving hospice care receive a psychiatric assessment—a study of psychosocial service provision within palliative care suggested that few hospices have access to psychiatric input (Lloyd-Williams *et al.* 1999).

Whilst it is acknowledged that some patients with depression may require expert psychiatric assessment, many patients can be adequately assessed by a doctor or nurse who has developed the necessary skills to do so. Ideally there should be an integrated referral system where patients can either be discussed or referred to a mental health-care professional and a plan of management initiated.

How can depression be assessed?

How can the doctor or nurse working in a palliative care unit establish that a patient is depressed and requires treatment or further assessment?

It would be justified to believe that patients should be able to describe their own symptoms but as discussed earlier many patients with advanced cancer are unwilling or unable to do so. Studies have also shown that patients underestimate their own distress and that asking an informant, for example, a close friend or relative is also unhelpful as their estimation of psychological distress is a closer measure of their own distress than that of the patient (Parkes 1985; Faller *et al.* 1995). Hoeper *et al.* (1984) found that physicians were influenced by the presence of a previous psychiatric history when making a diagnosis, showing a tendency to overdiagnose patients in whom a psychiatric diagnosis had previously been made. Hoeper also suggested that being screened for mental illness may prompt the patient to disclose more symptoms and concerns and could in itself be a therapeutic process.

One method of assessment is the use of rating scales. If we are to seek ways of improving the detection of psychiatric illness in the terminally ill population, there is a need to have rating scales with proven validity and established cut off thresholds.

The use of screening tools to assess for psychiatric morbidity has been advocated (Power *et al.* 1993). Such tools are not developed as diagnostic tools and can only serve to indicate whether a patient has particular psychiatric symptoms suggestive of a diagnosis of depression. The decision should then be taken whether to treat for depression or refer the patient for further assessment. Several instruments have been developed and researched with a particular score or cut-off threshold assigned in order to predict a 'case' of depression. The majority of rating scales consist of a number of symptoms or feelings on which the patient indicates their own response and the scores are calculated by the person administering the scale.

Many of these instruments have been developed and validated on physically healthy patients. Where an attempt has been made to validate instruments that would be used for patients with cancer, much work has been within the context of early disease or patients undergoing active treatment.

For screening tools to be of use, they must have validity, that is, does the scale actually measure what it is designed to measure? The assessment of validity is measured against a predetermined gold standard. There are several criteria of validity that should be achieved (Bowling 1997):

1. **Face validity.** Are the indicators or questions being used in the scale reasonable? Do they appear to be measuring what it has been claimed that they measuring? Is the scale relevant, reasonable, and acceptable for those who will be using the test?

2. **Content validity.** Do the components of the scale measure all aspects of the variable to be measured? Each item should reflect at least one of the content areas being measured. The number of items should reflect the importance given to each variable and be balanced.

3. **Criterion validity.** Can the variable be measured accurately? Can the scale be correlated with another measure, which is suitable and can be predefined as a 'gold standard'?

4. **Construct validity.** This is based on a theory or assumption of the associations and correlations of some items of the scale and is then examined to establish if they are correct. This is usually required when a gold standard test is not available.

A measurement scale or tool is tested for reliability, that is, does it give consistent results each time it is used with the same patient and are the results repeatable?

There is increasing interest in the use of screening scales within palliative care. The majority of rating scales consist of a number of symptoms or feelings on which the patient indicates their own response and and the scores are calculated by the person administering the scale.

Review of screening instruments available

The hospital anxiety and depression scale

The hospital anxiety and depression scale (HADS) is a 14-item scale that was devised in 1983 by Zigmond and Snaith for use with medical patients (Zigmond and Snaith 1983). Its main feature is that it excludes symptoms that may have both an emotional and physical aetiology, for example, change in appetite or sleep disturbance. It represents one of the most widely used depression-rating tools in cancer and palliative care.

The depression scale is based on anhedonia—the complete loss of enjoyment. Snaith (1992) described the concept of anhedonia as 'exclusion from the pleasure dome'. The authors of the scale stated that this symptom would indicate which patients may respond to anti-depressant medication (Snaith 1987). The HADS is now used extensively in Europe and the USA and has been translated into all European languages, Arabic, Japanese, Chinese, and Urdu.

Ramirez *et al.* (1995) screened patients with breast cancer during the first year after diagnosis and found that using a threshold total score of 11 in patients aged over 50 years, the HADS could identify women at risk from mood disorder in the year after diagnosis. Ibbotson *et al.* (1993) used the general health questionnaire (GHQ), the Rotterdam symptom checklist, and the HADS together with the psychiatric assessment schedule. Five hundred and thirteen patients were recruited. The HADS performed best in patients who were disease free or receiving active treatment using a cut-off threshold of greater than 19 in patients who were disease free.

Silverstone (1991) critically examined the concept of anhedonia in a psychiatric population using the HADS and found that anhedonia, which is measured by five of the seven items on the depression sub-scale, is present in 50 per cent of patients regardless of psychiatric disorder. He concluded that anhedonia is not pathognomic of a depressive disorder and cannot therefore be relied upon alone to differentiate depressive illness from other mental illness.

To ensure a scale can be usefully used within a population, it is important that a cut-off threshold is calculated and that this is validated against a predetermined gold standard. Examples of gold standards are a rigorous clinical interview or a method such as the present state examination—a semi-structured interview where responses are coded and by means of entry into a computer data program a psychiatric diagnosis can be obtained. A number of cut-off thresholds are selected and the thresholds analysed for sensitivity—the number of patients scoring at this threshold or above who are actually true cases, specificity—the number scoring below a threshold who are true non-cases, and the positive predictive value (ppv)—the probability that a score at the threshold or higher would be a true case.

Le Fevre (1999), in a study of the HADS and GHQ, concluded that the scores obtained on the anxiety and depression sub-scales should be summed rather than the depression sub-scale being used alone. A combined cut-off score of 20 gave a sensitivity of 77 per cent, a specificity of 85 per cent, and a ppv of 48 per cent. A further study (Lloyd-Williams *et al.* 2001) of 100 patients receiving palliative care with an estimated prognosis of six months or less found that the depression and anxiety sub-scales of the HADS showed poor efficacy for screening when used alone. The optimum threshold was at a combined cut-off of 19, which had a sensitivity of 68 per cent, a specificity of 67 per cent, and a ppv of 36 per cent. The authors also undertook individual item analysis of the HADS and found that the two items of the depression sub-scale that relate to subjective well-being and activity, that is, the item 'I still enjoy the things I used to enjoy' and the item 'I feel slowed down' were given a high score by the majority of patients. This suggests that these two items are poor discriminators for depression in patients with advanced metastatic disease. It is understandable why palliative care patients would respond positively to these questions due to their physical disease alone. It therefore appears from the above studies that the properties of the HADS and the symptoms it elicits have different discriminating power in those patients who have advanced metastatic cancer compared to those with early or stable disease.

The Edinburgh depression scale

This scale was devised by Cox *et al.* (1987, 1996) as a screening tool for postnatal depression. The scale contains 10 items and the items were selected to exclude the somatic symptoms of depression. The scale was devised so that healthcare workers with no prior knowledge of psychiatry could administer it. It is scored in the same format as the HADS, that is, the most negative response received the highest score. The original scale was validated on 84 mothers in the postnatal period and was found to have a sensitivity of 86 per cent and a specificity of 78 per cent using a cut-off threshold of 12/13. The authors believed it could be used for other populations but that the scale required validation prior to use. The scale contains questions concerning guilt, helplessness and hopelessness, subjective low mood, and thoughts of self-harm, which are thought to be particularly important diagnostic symptoms of depression in the terminally ill (Casey 1994).

Lloyd-Williams *et al.* (2000) compared the 10-item Edinburgh postnatal depression scale (EPDS) with a present state examination for depression according to the *International classification of diseases* (10th edn) criteria in 100 in-patients with metastatic cancer who were receiving palliative care. In this study a cut-off threshold of 13 gave an optimum sensitivity of 81 per cent, a specificity of 79 per cent, and a ppv of 53 per cent. The scale has since been used in other palliative care settings with favourable results (Taylor *et al.* in press). It appears therefore that a scale that was developed in a different context may well be useful as a screening tool for depression in patients with advanced cancer.

The general health questionnaire

The GHQ and the standardized psychiatric interview were used among 126 consecutive patients admitted to an oncology ward (Hardman *et al.* 1988). The GHQ consists of a checklist of statements asking respondents to indicate their response on a four-point scale. The GHQ identified 79 per cent of affective disorders and 34 per cent false positives (medical and nursing staff only correctly identified 49 per cent of patients). Le Fevre *et al.* (1999) administered the HADS and the 12-item GHQ (GHQ-12) to 79 hospice in-patients (all except one were suffering from advanced cancer) and compared them with diagnoses generated from a revised clinical interview schedule. The GHQ-12 was adapted from the original 60-item GHQ and was designed to give a general indication of psychiatric 'caseness' rather than a specific diagnosis of depression. The results show that in the palliative care in-patient population the HADS appears to perform better than the GHQ-12 in identifying cases fulfilling Endicott diagnostic criteria for depression. The authors' postulate that this may be because the GHQ-12 contains questions on somatic symptoms—they do not give sensitivities and specificities for the GHQ-12 scale.

Beck depression inventory

The Beck depression inventory (Beck *et al.* 1961) consists of 21 items each with a four-point scale response and the items are summated to achieve a score. This scale was devised and initially validated for use with psychiatric patients, has suggested cut-off thresholds for both research and clinical use, and is widely used in research. A short form of the Beck, which consists of 13 items, has been developed as a screening tool for use with medical patients and has been found to correlate well with the longer version (Beck and Beck 1972). The Beck is widely used in medical settings. Chochinov *et al.* (1997) assessed 197 palliative care in-patients with advanced cancer using the 13-item short form of the Beck. Using a recommended cut-off score of eight on the Beck, a sensitivity of 79 per cent, a specificity of 71 per cent, and a ppv of 27 per cent were achieved.

The Zung self-rating depression scale

The Zung self rating scale (Zung 1967) is a 20-item self-report measure of the symptoms of depression and patients rate their symptoms according to how they have felt the previous week. Scores are categorized into four different levels according to the patient's indication of the presence or absence of symptoms and these four levels suggest the presence or absence of depressive symptoms. As with all screening tools it does not yield a diagnosis but indicates whether patients have levels of clinical symptoms that may be suggestive of a depressive illness. The Zung scale and the briefer 11-item Zung scale, which excludes nine items relating to somatic symptoms, has been used in cancer patients (predominantly those with stable disease) and found to be a useful screening tool (Dugan *et al.* 1998; Passik *et al.* 2000).

Other methods of assessment—visual analogue scales and asking 'Are you depressed?'

Visual analogue scales have been used in psychiatric patients (Luria 1975), in patients with stroke (House *et al.* 1989), and in patients with cancer (Coates *et al.* 1983) but the subjective experience of the patient may lead to either under- or overscoring. Lees *et al.* (1999) found that despite the apparent simplicity of this method more than 50 per cent of patients admitted to a hospice during the study period were unable to complete the visual analogue scale and although careful explanation was given as to how the visual analogue scale should be completed, many patients did not understand what was required of them when asked to indicate their mood on a 100 mm visual analogue scale.

Mahoney *et al.* (1994) and Chochinov *et al.* (1997) suggested asking patients if they are depressed was a useful indicator as to whether patients may be depressed. Chochinov *et al.* assessed 197 palliative care in-patients with advanced cancer using four screening tools together with a diagnostic interview for depression according to research diagnostic criteria. The diagnostic interview was adapted from the schedule for affective disorders and schizophrenia (SADS). The 13-item short form of the Beck depression inventory was developed as a rapid screening technique for use with medical patients. A single question assessing depressed mood ('Are you depressed?'), taken from the full SADS interview, correctly identified the eventual diagnostic outcome of every patient with a sensitivity, a specificity, and a ppv of 100 per cent suggesting that asking this single question could be a diagnostic test. Extending the screening interview by adding a second question assessing loss of interest reduced the specificity to 98 per cent but not the sensitivity, which remained at 100 per cent; ppv was

86 per cent. However recent research carried out in the UK (Taylor *et al.* in press), using the single question against a clinical psychiatric interview, found that the single question had a sensitivity and specificity of less than 60 per cent suggesting that further work may be required before advocating the widespread use of this question as a screening tool.

Depression and thoughts of self-harm

Although by no means diagnostic, thoughts of self-harm are important predictors of depression in the terminally ill patient and when carrying out any form of psychiatric interview or screening with terminally ill patients, it is appropriate to enquire whether they have suicidal thoughts. Many palliative care staff believe that self-harm and suicide are rare events among the palliative care population but this is not the case; the study of Grzybowska and Finlay (1997) reported 21 suicides and 37 attempted suicides in a five-year period in hospices within the UK. Women cancer patients are nearly twice as likely and men cancer patients 1.3 times more likely to die of suicide than the general population (Louhivori and Hakama 1979) and a far higher than expected number of suicides occur in patients with malignant disease (Whitlock 1978). In a recent UK study of 248 patients with advanced cancer, 30 per cent reported thoughts of self-harm at some point in the previous seven days and patients who reported thoughts of self harm were found to be significantly younger (Lloyd-Williams in press).

An overwhelming feeling of helplessness and hopelessness has previously been reported as an indicator of suicidal risk (Kovacs *et al.* 1975) and such symptoms are also commonly found in patients who are depressed.

Brown *et al.* (1986) and Chochinov *et al.* (1995) reported that the presence of suicidal thoughts and desire for death were almost exclusively linked to the presence of a psychiatric disorder in the terminally ill patient.

Brown *et al.* (1986) assessed desire for death as part of a psychiatric interview and looked at the association with scores of the Beck depression inventory and with a diagnosis of clinical depression based on a psychiatric structured interview using the third edition of the *Diagnostic and statistical manual of mental disorders* (*DSM-III*) criteria. Desire for death and suicidal ideas were found exclusively in those who were found to be clinically depressed.

Chochinov *et al.* (1995) looked at desire for death as part of a structured psychiatric interview in 200 patients admitted to the palliative care units of two hospitals. The Beck depression inventory was also used, as were measures of performance status, pain, and social support. Desire for death and suicidal ideas were found exclusively in those who were found to be clinically depressed. Association was identified between desire for death and the diagnosis of clinical depression ($P=0.09$) and depression emerged as the only factor that independently predicted desire for death in the study population. It is essential therefore that patients who are thought to be depressed are asked about thoughts of self-harm. Staff may find this a difficult subject to broach; a possible question would be 'Have you ever felt so sad that you wished you could do something to end your life?'. Patients who have had such thoughts frequently express relief at being asked about them and being able to share their thoughts and feelings.

When should patients be screened?

Many professionals working in palliative care are concerned that screening for depression may not be appropriate in a population of patients whose illness is changing rapidly, but a recent study revealed that patient scores on a validated scale (EDS) were remarkably stable. All patients referred to and attending a palliative care day unit were invited to participate in a 12-week study. Fifty patients participated and the scores of all patients who scored below the cut-off threshold at initial assessment showed a mean change of ±0.56 (range −6 to +7) on the screening tool. In only three patients did the scores change over the time period from below to above the threshold. The test–re-test reliability was calculated and kappa was 0.767, suggesting that these findings were real and not due to frequent testing (Riddleston and Lloyd-Williams in press). This study suggested that screening palliative care patients for depression at referral or first assessment may be useful in assessing depression within the palliative care setting. It is crucial however to remain as vigilant for new symptoms suggesting depression as for new physical symptoms.

Why diagnose depression in the terminally ill?

Depression is the most common psychiatric illness in patients with terminal cancer. Patients who are depressed may also have physical symptoms that are difficult to palliate and that may improve as their depression is appropriately treated. Psychological and psychiatric morbidity can be a major source of distress to terminally ill patients and to their relatives and friends. There are many anti-depressants available with acceptable side-effect profiles and patients identified as depressed even within the last four to six weeks of life may still benefit from treatment. This emphasizes the importance of diagnosis. Valid cut-off thresholds on self-assessment tools may be a useful aid in the process of diagnosis. The availability of appropriate psychosocial expertise is also necessary to provide optimum care for terminally ill patients who develop symptoms of depression.

Conclusions

If we are to improve the diagnosis of depression in palliative care patients, depression needs to be given the same attention as physical symptoms, for example, pain, breathlessness, or vomiting. Patients may be unwilling or unable to describe their symptoms of depression and therefore it is important that staff are aware of its high prevalence and know how to elicit the symptoms. Screening tools may have a role in the assessment of depression in this population and tools such as the HADS, the EDPS, the GHQ-12, and the single question 'Are you depressed' have been validated for this population (Lloyd-Williams *et al.* in press) (Table 7.1) . Care however needs to be taken to ensure that patients are not diagnosed on the basis of obtaining a certain score. Assessment of depression requires sensitive questioning as to the patient's own perception of their mood together with questions on other areas, for example, excessive or inappropriate guilt, hopelessness, helplessness, and thoughts of self-harm or suicide.

Table 7.1 Screening Tools for Depression

Tool	Cut-off score	Population	Diagnostic criteria	Sensitivity	Specificity	ppv
One-item question (Chochinov)	N/A	197 in-patients with advanced cancer	RDC	100%	100%	100%
Two-item question (Chochinov)	N/A	197 in-patients with advanced cancer	RDC	100%	98%	86%
Edinburgh postnatal depression scale (Lloyd-Williams)	13	100 palliative care in-patients with metastatic cancer	ICD-10	81%	79%	53%
Hospital anxiety and depression scale (Le Fevre)	20 combined	79 palliative care in-patients	Endicott	77%	85%	48%
Visual analogue scale (Chochinov)	55 mm	197 in-patients with advanced cancer	RDC	72%	50%	17%

N/A, not applicable; RDC, Research Diagnostic Criteria; ICD-10, International Classification of Diseases (10th edition).

References

Addington-Hall J, McCarthy M (1995). Dying from cancer: results of a national population-based investigation. *Palliative Med* 9:295–305.

American Psychiatric Association (1994). *Diagnostic and statistical manual of mental disorders.* Washington, DC: American Psychiatric Association.

Barraclough J (1994). *Cancer and emotion.* Radcliffe Medical Press.

Beck A, Beck R (1972). Screening depressed patients in family practice: a rapid technique. *Postgrad Med* 52:81–5.

Beck A, Ward C, Mendelson M, Mock J, Erbaugh J (1961). An inventory of measuring depression. *Arch Gen Psychiat* 4:562–71.

Bergevin P, Bergevin R (1995). Recognising depression. *Am J Hospice Palliative Care* 12:22–3.

Block S (2000). Assessing and managing depression in the terminally ill patient. *Ann Intern Med* 132:209–18.

Bowling A (1997). *Measuring health—a review of quality of life instruments.* Buckingham: Open University Press.

Brietbart W, Bruera E, Chochinov H, Lynch M (1995). Neuropsychiatric syndromes and psychological symptoms in patients with advanced cancer. *J Pain Sympt Manage* 1995; 10:131–41.

Brown J, Henteleff P, Barakat S, Rowe C (1986). Is it normal for terminally ill patients to desire death? *Am J Psychiat* 143:208–11.

Brugha T (1993). Depression in the terminally ill. *Br J Hosp Med* 1993; 50:175–81.

Buckberg J, Penman D, Holland J (1984). Depression in hospitalised cancer patients. *Psychosomat Med* 1984; **46**:199–211.

Casey P (1994). Depression in the dying—disorder or distress. *Prog Palliative Care* **2**:1–3.

Cavanaugh S (1984). Diagnosing depression in the hospitalised patient with chronic medical illness. *J Clin Psychiat* **45**:13–16.

Chochinov H, Wilson K, Enns M, Lander S (1994). Prevalence of depression in the terminally ill: effects of diagnostic criteria and symptom threshold judgements. *Am J Psychiat* **151**:537–40.

Chochinov H, Wilson K, Enns M, Mouton N, Landau S, Levitate M *et al.* (1995). Desire for death in the terminally ill. *Am J Psychiat* **152**:1185–91.

Chochinov H, Wilson K, Enns M, Lander S (1997). Are you depressed ? Screening for depression in the terminally ill. *Am J Psychiat* **154**:674–6.

Coates A, Dillnebeck C, McNeil D, Kaye S, Sims K, Fox R *et al.* (1983). On the receiving end—11. Linear analogue self assessment (LASA) in evaluation of aspects of the quality of life of cancer patients receiving therapy. *Eur J Cancer Clin Oncol* **19**:1633–7.

Cox J, Holden J, Sagovsky R (1987). Detection of postnatal depression: development of 10 item Edinburgh Postnatal Depression Scale. *Br J Psychiat* **150**:782–6.

Cox J, Chapman G, Murray D, Jones P (1996). Validation of the Edinburgh postnatal scale (EPDS) in non-postnatal women. *J Affect Disord* **39**:185–9.

Dugan W, McDonald M, Passik S, Rosenfield B, Theobald D, Edgerton S (1998). Use of Zung self-rating depression scale in cancer patients: feasibility as a screening tool. *Psycho-oncology* **7**:483–93.

Endicott J (1984). Measurement of depression in patients with cancer. *Cancer* **53**:2243–8.

Faller H, Lang H, Schilling S (1995). Emotional distress and hope in lung cancer patients, as perceived by patients, relatives, physicians, nurses and interviewers. *Psycho-oncology* **4**:21–31.

Fulton C (1997). The physical and psychological symptoms experienced by patients with metastatic breast cancer before death. *Eur J Cancer Care* **6**:262–6.

Grzybowska P, Finlay I (1997). The incidence of suicide in palliative care patients. *Palliative Med* **11**:313–16.

Haig R (1992). Management of depression in patients with advanced cancer. *Med J Austral* **156**:499–503.

Hardman A, Maguire P, Crowther D (1988). The recognition of psychiatric morbidity on a medical oncology ward. *J Psychosomat Res* **33**:235–9.

Hinton J (1963). The physical and mental distress of the dying. *Q J Med* **32**:1–21.

Hoeper E, Kessler L, Pierce W , Nycz G, Burke J (1984). Screening for mental illness. *Lancet* **1**(8377):635–6.

House A, Dennis M, Hawton K, Warlow C (1989). Methods of identifying mood disorders in stroke patients: experience in the Oxfordshire community Stroke Project. *Age Ageing* **18**:371–9.

Hughes J (1985) Depressive illness and lung cancer. II Follow-up of inoperable patients. *Eur J Surg Oncol* **11**:21–4.

Ibbotson T, Maguire P, Selby T, Priestman T, Wallace L (1993). Screening for anxiety and depression in cancer patients:the effects of disease and treatment. *Eur J Cancer* **30**:37–40.

International Classification of mental and behavioural disorders (1992). Geneva: WHO.

Kovacs M, Beck A, Weissman A (1975). Hoplessness; an indicator of suicidal risk. *Suicide* **5**:98–103.

Lees N, Lloyd-Williams M (1999). Assessing depression in palliative care patients using the visual analogue scale: a pilot study. *Eur J Cancer Care* 8:220–3.

Le Fevre P, Devereux J, Smith S, Lawrie SM, Cornbleet M (1999). Screening for psychiatric illness in the palliative care inpatient setting: a comparison between the Hospital Anxiety and Depression Scale and the General Health Questionnaire-12. *Palliative Med* 12:399–407.

Lloyd-Williams M (2002). How common are thoughts of self harm in a UK palliative care population? *Support Care Cancer* 10:422–24.

Lloyd-Williams M, Friedman T, Rudd N (1999). A survey of psychosocial servuce provision within hospices. *Palliative Med* 13:431–2.

Lloyd-Williams M, Friedman T, Rudd N (2000). Criterion validation of the Edinburgh Postnatal Depression Scale as a screening tool for depression in patients with advanced metastatic cancer. *J Pain Sympt Manage* 20:259–65.

Lloyd-Williams M, Friedman T, Rudd N (2001). An analysis of the validity of the of the Hospital Anxiety and Depression scale as a screening tool in patients with advanced metastatic cancer. *J Pain Sympt Manage* 22:990–6.

Lloyd-Williams M, Spiller J, Ward J (2003). Which screening tools should be used to screen palliative care patients for depression? *Palliative Med.*

Louhivori K, Hakama M (1979). Risk of suicide among cancer patients. *Am J Epidemiol* 109:59–65.

Luria R (1975). The validity and reliability of the visual analogue mood scale. *J Psychiat Res* 12:51–7.

Maguire P (1985). Improving the detection of psychiatric problems in cancer patients. *Soc Sci Med* 20:819–23.

Maguire P, Howell A (1995). Improving the psychological care of cancer patients In: Houses A, Mayou R, Mallinson C (ed.). *Psychiatric aspects of physical disease.* London: Royal college of Physicians and Royal College of Psychiatrists. pp. 41–54.

Mahoney J, Drinka T, Abler R, Gunter-Hunt G, Matthews C, Gravenstein S *et al.* (1994). Screening for depression: single question versus GDS. *J Am Geriat Soc* 42:1006–8.

McVey P (1998). Depression among the palliative care oncology population. *Int J Palliative Nursing* 4:86–93.

Parkes CM (1985). Terminal care: home, hospital or hospice? *Lancet* 1(8421):155 –7.

Pasacreta J, Massie M (1990). Nurses reports of psychiatric complications in patients with cancer. *Oncol Nurses Forum* 17:347–53.

Passik S, Lundberg J, Rosenfield B, Kirsh K, Donaghy K, Theobald D *et al.* (2000). Factor analysis of the Zung self-rating depression scale in a large ambulatory oncology sample. *Psychosomatics* 41:121–7.

Power D, Kelly S, Gilsenan J, Kearney M, O'Mahony D, Walsh J *et al.* (1993). Suitable screening tests for cognitive impairment and depression in the terminally ill—a prospective prevalence study. *Palliative Med* 7:213–18.

Ramirez A, Richards M, Jarrett S, Fnetiman I (1995). Can mood disorder in women with breast cancer be identified preoperatively? *Br J Cancer* 72:1509–12.

Ramsay N (1992). Referral to a liaison psychiatrist from a palliative care unit. *Palliative Med* 16:54–60.

Riddleston H, Lloyd-Williams M (2003). When should palliative care patients be screened for depression. *J Pain Sympt Manage.*

Silverstone P (1991). Is anhedonia a good measure of depression? *Acta Psychiat Scand* **83**:249–50.

Snaith P (1992). Anhedonia: exclusion from the pleasure dome. *BMJ* **305**:134.

Snaith P (1987). The concepts of mild depression. *Br J Psychiat* **150**:387–93.

Taylor F, Lloyd-Williams M, Dennis M (in press). Is asking UK palliative care patients the single question "are you depressed?" a robust method of screening for depression? *Br J Psychiat.*

Valentine S, Saunders J (1989). Dealing with serious depression in cancer patients. *Nursing* 44–7.

Whitlock F (1978). Suicide, cancer and depression. *Br J Psychiat* **132**:269–74.

Zigmond AS, Snaith RP (1983). The Hospital Anxiety and Depression Scale. *Acta Psychiat Scand* **67**:361–70.

Zung W (1967). Factors influencing the self-rating depression scale. *Arch Gen Psychiat* **16**:543–47.

Chapter 8

Psychosocial care for non-malignant disease

Rod MacLeod

Introduction

The principles and practice of palliative care make no mention of any disease-specific approaches and yet historically it is people who have malignant disease who make up the largest cohort of those receiving this approach to care. The report of the US Institute of Medicine (Approaching death: improving care at the end of life, Field and Cassel 1997) begins 'Humane care for those approaching death is a social obligation as well as a personal offering from those directly involved'. Care, both in terms of attending to a patient's physical needs and their psychological well-being, may have social and personal motivations and there is nothing to suggest that there should be any difference in the mode or way of caring that is dependent on the diagnosis of the person who is dying (Table 8.1).

Various theories exploring the concept of care have attributed to it a sense of social or moral obligation. A humanistic model of caring is characterized by the sense that caring is a moral obligation, a mode of being that calls for a philosophy of moral commitment to protecting human dignity. This is the type of caring that health professionals are called on for and expected to provide; it is a caring created by the obligation to provide good (MacLeod 2000). Not only is caring a moral orientation but also it incorporates the attributes of honesty, respect, and trustworthiness into all aspects of moral behaviour (Branch 2000). Yet aside from the notion of moral obligation, the concept of care also concerns what the US Institute of Medicine calls a 'personal offering'. The caring person listens, responds, and relates to the patient as a unique individual, attempting to understand the other's needs and feelings (Kutner *et al.* 1999; Watson 1988) Care can begin when one individual enters into the lifeworld of another person and attempts to understand what it is like to be that person.

In his book *The illness narratives*, Kleinman (1988) outlines his understanding of how the interpretation of illness meanings or narratives can contribute to more effective care. He sets out a practical clinical method that practitioners can (and should) apply to provide more effective and humane care (of chronically sick people). He writes that this

> alternative therapeutic approach originates in the reconceptualization of medical care as (1) empathic witnessing of the existential experience of suffering and (2) practical coping with the major psychosocial crises that constitute the menacing chronicity of that experience. The work of the practitioner includes the sensitive soliciting of the patient's and the family's stories of the illness, the assembling of a mini-ethnography of the changing concepts of chronicity, informed negotiation with alternative lay perspectives on care, and what amounts to brief psychotherapy for the multiple, ongoing threats and losses that make chronic illness [and terminal illness] so profoundly disruptive.

He concludes by stating that not the least of the reasons for studying the illness meanings, therefore, is that such an investigation can help the patient, the family, and also the practitioner: certainly not every time, perhaps not even routinely, but often enough to make a significant difference.

He contends that ultimately what the practitioner does best is to organize care around the phenomenological appreciation of the illness experience and its psychological and social consequences for the patient.

Kleinman also expands on the development of his rationale for a practical clinical methodology in the care of the chronically ill but this also has particular relevance for the care of people who are dying from non-malignant diseases who have often experienced the relentless chronicity of, say, end-organ failure. The essence of that methodology is captured in the words empathic listening, translation, and interpretation. By translation and interpretation he means the affirmation of the patient's experience of illness as constituted by lay explanatory models and to negotiate an acceptable therapeutic approach. Another core clinical task is the empathic interpretation of a life story into the subject matter of a biography (placing the illness in the context of the lifeworld of that particular individual and their family).

Much of what he writes about is removed from the classical medical model of care but has a bearing on the provision of psychosocial care for people at the end of life.

Psychosocial care, as identified by a discussion document from the National Council for Hospice and Specialist Palliative Care Services (1997), includes psychological approaches concerned with enabling the patient and those close to them to express thoughts, feelings, and concerns relating to illness. It also focuses on assessing their individual needs and resources and ensuring that psychological and emotional support is available. That document goes on to define psychosocial interventions as those interventions by health professionals (or occasionally trained volunteers) using psychological methods intended to improve the psychological and emotional well-being of the patient and their family. Such interventions include counselling and psychotherapy, behavioural and cognitive techniques, and educational therapies such as training and coping skills and providing information to enhance the patient's sense of control.

Psychosocial support means care which does not use formal psychological methods but enhances well-being, confidence, and social functioning. This would include support groups and befriending or visiting schemes.

Table 8.1

Care is a personal offering as well as a moral obligation

There is a well-established need for psychosocial care for people who are dying from non-malignant diseases

Information about those needs is often lacking in referral information to palliative care teams

Predicting life expectancy in non-cancer patients is problematic

The needs of all dying people are similar

There is

a physical context

a spiritual context

a social context

an emotional context

a psychological context

a cultural context

a sexual context

Remaining in charge of their living is important near the end of life for most people

Maintaining hope, creativity, quality of life, and dignity are paramount

Education is the key to effective care for people who are with non-malignant disease

---

Whilst it is generally acknowledged that there is a well-established need for psychosocial care for people with non-malignant disease there is surprisingly little attention paid to this in the literature. It is estimated that almost 72 000 people who die from non-malignant disease in England and Wales each year may require specialist palliative care (Addington-Hall *et al.* 1998)—this represents almost 17 per cent of people who died in the regional study of care for the dying. This figure suggestss that there would be a 79 per cent increase in case load if specialist palliative care services were made fully available to non-cancer patients. That study identified that referral criteria were different for people with cancer and with non-malignant disease, in that those with non-malignant disease were, on average, older and they also had different patterns of dependency. Symptom management is a cornerstone of palliative care—the data suggests that a sixth of people with non-malignant disease had similar levels of symptom 'load' to the most severely affected third of cancer patients. No specific mention is made in that study of the psychosocial aspects of care that were required—and therein lies part of the problem. Whilst the focus of much in palliative care is on the relief of physical symptoms there are equal, if not greater, burdens to be relieved in non-physical management.

A retrospective review identified the pattern of non-cancer referrals to a specialist palliative care service (Kite *et al.* 1999)—29 per cent of the hospital ward referrals had a non-cancer diagnosis. They were referred predominantly for symptom control. Of 130 out-patient referrals 23 per cent had a non-cancer diagnosis and again were also predominantly referred for the management of pain. Nine per cent of 196 home care referrals had a non-cancer diagnosis. They tended to be referred for 'multiprofessional care' of end-stage disease. Only 4 per cent of 421 hospice in-patient admissions were for patients with a non-cancer diagnosis and were predominantly for respite care.

Massarotto *et al.* (2000), in a study of the information provided by hospital referrers to a hospice, showed that 60 per cent of doctors provided information on the patient's living situation. Other psychological, spiritual, and social support information such as the patient's emotional state, adequacy of support, the family's problems in relation to the illness, and cultural and religious affiliations were poorly documented with generally less than 10 per cent of referrers providing this information. This could be explained by such factors as a limitation on their time to prepare referral letters, a general lack of emphasis by doctors as a discipline on the patient's non-medical needs, and a lack of day-to-day contact with patients. These deficiencies could be a result of, or lead to, inadequate knowledge of their psychological, social, and spiritual needs.

'If there is a case for palliative care in cancer, the ethical case of palliative care beyond cancer is resounding and restricted practice is indefensible.' George and Sykes (1997) identify a number of practical problems with facilities and approaches to the provision of palliative care for people with non-malignant disease.

1. Patients severely incapacitated through slowly progressive disease require much personal attention and may also require specialized equipment and skills.

2. The prognosis in these patients is usually less clear-cut than with cancer.

3. The integration of non-cancer patients into palliative care facilities for those with cancer has been controversial, for example, Alzheimer's disease.

The philosophy of care for these groups however, is quite the same. It is not reductive but divergent, exploring all aspects of each individual's world in order to identify and begin to understand each person's suffering, pain, or distress.

How then can current models of palliative care be extended to non-cancer patients? There are certain elements that are the same whatever the nature of disease. Information needs, high levels of psychological distress, and carer distress are all fundamental aspects of care for people who are dying. Firstly though, it may be helpful to try to identify some of the elements that are deemed to be different in the care of people with cancer and those with non-malignant disease.

Field (1998) identified two important differences between patients with cancer and those with non-malignant conditions. First, differences in disease progression mean there is a continuing benefit from curative and restorative interventions and treatments for the latter category. Second, there is greater uncertainty about the fact and likely time of death with non-cancer patients. He identifies the latter as appearing to be the key obstruction to extending specialist palliative care services to non-cancer patients. This is because they will not be seen as suitable candidates for palliative care until they have been defined as terminally ill. One of the reasons that this may occur is because of the difficulty many clinicians have in dealing with uncertainty in general. In medicine, and possibly in other disciplines as well, uncertainty stimulates and propels activity (Hall 2002)—doctors have a 'propensity to resolve uncertainty and ambiguity by action rather than inaction' (Katz 1984). Increasing diagnostic uncertainty leads to a reluctance to withdraw from 'active' interventions so leaving patients and families in a similar situation of ambiguity and doubt about the future (Christakis and Asch 1993). There is evidence from the study to understand prognoses and preferences for outcomes and risks of treatments (SUPPORT) (SUPPORT Principal Investigators 1996) suggesting widespread difficulty in predicting the life expectancy of hospitalized non-cancer patients. This relates to a tendency for the continuation of what might be deemed futile treatment in the face of relentlessly advancing disease. Taken out of context (that is, without considering the person as a whole) almost any disease may be deemed 'treatable'—such are the advances in medical science and technology. This confidence in the advancement of medical science is relayed not only to the medical and nursing professions but to the lay public as well, with a consequent sense of expectation that is unfortunately not wholly realized. This situation is compounded with the advancing age of people being treated. Many elderly patients have multiple clinical diagnoses involving multi-system pathology and the diagnosis of dying is often made only by exclusion. Communication may be more difficult due to a combination of a higher incidence of confusion in elderly patients with non-malignant disease than in younger cancer patients and reduced social networks in the elderly may lead to reduced care and support from family and friends. It is claimed that the diagnosis of dying is more difficult in elderly people (Seale 1991). The incidence, duration, intensity, and type of symptoms follow a different pattern in cancer compared to other illnesses. It is also suggested that long-term mental confusion and disability, as well as other symptoms related to age, are more common in non-cancer patients, who also tend to be older, and people aged 75 and over who do not die from cancer are more likely to have outlasted their spouses, brothers, and sisters and even their children. They are predominantly women and many live alone or in residential care.

Nevertheless, the psychosocial aspects of care of the dying person, whatever their diagnosis, include the need for

(1) understanding—of symptoms and the nature of disease and of the process of dying;

(2) acceptance—regardless of mood, sociability, and appearance;

(3) self-esteem—involvement in decision making;

(4) safety—a feeling of security;

(5) belonging—a wish to feel needed and not to feel a burden;

(6) love—expressions of affection and human contact (touch);

(7) spirituality—an explanation of meaning and purpose, both religious and non-religious;

(8) hope—for an improvement in any aspect of their life or of their living.

In the provision of psychosocial care for people at the end of life each of these needs must be identified and addressed.

Social context

Dying from a non-malignant disease, in many ways, takes on a different social structure or standing than dying from cancer. The language that we use is quite different—for example people who die from cancer are often referred to as 'brave' in their 'battle' with cancer. They often talk of 'beating' the disease or 'fighting' it. Non-malignant disease does not seem to have that same social cache. Death from end-organ failure is often silent and slow—in many ways relentless in its nature. Without heroic medical interventions to replace organs or use artificial means to support ailing bodies many of these people would die earlier and perhaps more suddenly. In identifying social or psychological care for these people it is important to recognize this significant difference in perception of disease, which may have originated both from the individual and society.

For many people with cancer there are well-recognized social networks or programmes that may provide both psychological and social support. Social support for people with non-malignant diseases should emerge from people in similar situations, family and friends, and the wider community. Many of the current support systems for people with non-malignant disease are focused on raising awareness and funding for curative interventions rather than supporting people in the last stages of their disease. The professions, whilst openly supporting cancer networks and programmes, have been slower to acknowledge the need for similar systems for people with incurable non-malignant disease.

Emotional context

Nevertheless, there are feelings and emotions that are almost universally experienced near the end of life.

1. Fear of being left alone or having to leave loved ones, of breaking down or losing control, and of the situation they are currently in, getting worse.
2. A sense of helplessness in which physical and psychological crises show up human powerlessness. Alongside this is the knowledge of physical and emotional strength gradually deteriorating, loss of physical ability bringing with it attendant psychological and social helplessness.
3. Feelings of sadness for what is not to be and for the loss to come.
4. A sense of longing for all that has gone before and all that is not going to be, in the future.
5. Feelings of guilt for being better off than others or regret for things that have been done or not done.
6. A sense of shame for having been exposed as helpless, emotional, needing others, or not having reacted as one would have wished.
7. Anger at what has happened, at whatever caused it or allowed it to happen, that the treatment has not worked, at the injustice and senselessness of it all, at the shame and indignity, and at the lack of proper understanding by others.

These feelings and emotions may also be influenced by memories of feelings or loss or of love for other people in their lives who have been injured or died, perhaps let down by doctors, by the system, or by the family.

Psychological context

Many or all of these feelings may be identified during a more formal psychological evaluation of the patient and family (Fisher 1995).

Initially it is helpful to look for indicators of pathological levels of psychological disturbance such as clinical depression or other mood disturbance or personality disorders. These lend themselves well to specific psychological interventions. Variables suggesting that the patient or family are at serious risk of psychological disorder or distress may be identified (for example, social isolation or a history of psychiatric hospitalizations). All members of the healthcare team may observe and subjectively report distress that they feel is psychological in nature (fear or anger) or psychologically mediated (pain or breathlessness) but may not meet the criteria of a discrete psychological disorder. The team should also look for the potential for preventative interventions that may forestall, minimize, or bolster resources for predictable areas or times of vulnerability and hardship (similar patterns of ill-health, prebereavement work, or anniversary calls to the bereaved).

Specific psycho-educational interventions that may enhance coping skills, psychological insights, and quality of life should be employed, regardless of the presence or absence of clinical levels of psychological distress.

People with neuromuscular degenerative disorders such as motor neurone disease (MND), multiple sclerosis (MS), and muscular dystrophies and less frequent disorders like Creutzfeldt–Jacob disease may have particular psychological needs associated with their care. Such disorders bring with them potentially challenging communication issues. For example, some patients may not be able to communicate verbally but retain effective cognitive functioning (Oneschuk 2001). It is important to help families to differentiate between behavioural disturbances associated with cognitive impairment and other communication difficulties. Cognitive impairment, depressive symptoms, emotional incontinence, or lability all need expert assessment and careful explanation and management. All or any of these may significantly impact on coping ability, psychological adjustment, and communication both of the patient and the family (Macleod 2001).

Cultural context

In palliative care the cornerstone of practice is the holistic approach to care that is exemplified by the management of 'total' pain. This classically includes physical, psychological, social, and spiritual pain. Cultural pain or distress can be expressed through any of these dimensions (Oliviere 1999). Often closely allied to culture are spiritual and religious beliefs that have a bearing on how people approach and understand their disease. In many societies people define themselves by their religious, cultural, or tribal grouping, even when their faith or immersion in religion or culture is limited. There are wide variations between people of differing faiths, ethnic backgrounds, and national origins and their approach to the end of life. Although documented evidence is thin there is anecdotal evidence to suggest that there is a difference in approach to dealing with malignant and non-malignant disease. In order to understand these differences it is important to understand the culture from the perspective of the patient and family. Cultural safety was a term originally identified by a New Zealand nursing scholar, Irihapeti Ramsden, that became incorporated into guidelines for nurses and midwives in training in that country. The concept of cultural safety states that (Nursing Council 1996)

> the effective nursing of a person/family from another culture recognises the impact of the nurse's culture on his or her practice. Unsafe clinical practice is any action which diminishes, demeans or disempowers the cultural identity and wellbeing of an individual.

Cultural safety is now a concept that is identified and embraced in all healthcare practices throughout New Zealand and in many other parts of the world. In the management of non-malignant disease it is helpful to identify any particular taboos or discrimination that people may experience as a result of their diagnosis (for example, AIDS or neuromuscular disorders) (Department of Health 1987).

In caring for people of a different culture to our own it is imperative that we understand the expectations of that culture in order that we act appropriately (Kashiwagi 1995). Without the accurate and honest provision of information in the right form, at the right time, there can be little hope of an understanding being reached about the situation the patient and family are facing and the goals of care that are being formulated. Without asking, we cannot know what individuals need to make a difference to the end of their life. That asking must include an acknowledgement of difference—difference in culture, in religious beliefs, in understanding of the nature of disease, in expectations in a particular situation, and in perceptions for hope at the end of life. Professionals must remain honest and open at all times—'truth is like a drug and has its own pharmacology; insufficient doses are ineffective and may harm the patient's trust in the therapist'.

Sexual context

Sexuality is an element of being that is often easily sidelined or overlooked when caring for people at the end of life, particularly if those people are elderly. It is too often assumed that because people approaching death are weak and tired that their sexual needs are minimized but this fails to recognize the many ways in which human beings can express their sexuality aside form sexual intercourse. Staff often view people's sexual interests as 'behavioural problems' rather than natural occurrences or expressions of needs for loving contact (Steinke 1997; McPherson et al. 2001). Many people approaching the end of life with a non-malignant disease have had a relentless decrease in their physical being for some time. Much of their time may have been spent in repeated hospital admissions and the physical isolation that encourages. Many treatments, as well as the diseases themselves, can affect sexual performance and of course sexual activity may not be at the forefront of people's minds as they approach death. Acknowledging that all people are sexual beings is a starting point in helping people address their sexual needs and wishes—it is in no way different from acknowledging that they are physical or emotional beings. Taking a sexual health history may be one way of ensuring this aspect of each individual's being is not overlooked. This is one aspect of their functional health that can contribute to their sense of self-worth or self-esteem. Changes in physical appearance, size, and skin colour and texture as well as increasing fatigue often decrease an individual's sense of self-worth or attractiveness. Identifying psychological elements of their functional health may help to reverse this decrease. Providing information and advice on ways of expressing sexuality other than through sexual intercourse may help to restore an individual's sense of worth in this aspect of themselves.

Remaining in charge

A recent study confirmed the importance of remaining 'in charge' whilst living with a terminal illness. Whilst respondents in that study all had malignant disease, earlier work suggested similar themes and patterns that were evident from people living with chronic disabling conditions. Each of five themes focused on life and living in relation to life as it was or would be without illness. Both practical issues of daily living and the opportunity to address philosophical issues surrounding the meaning and purpose of life emerged as important areas in both groups. These themes were related and interconnected—both influencing and being influenced by one another. These studies confirm what may seem to be an obvious truism; that is, the way in which health professionals manage patients' involvement in areas of symptom management can impact on areas of existential concern. Similarly therefore, areas of psychological or social concern may well impact negatively on physical well-being.

Establishing and understanding the patient's perspective in relation to these themes may assist health professionals in developing management strategies most appropriate to the individual patient's needs.

The maintenance of hope

A review of health professionals' perceptions of hope (MacLeod *et al.* in press; MacLeod and Carter 1999) reconfirmed that hope is central to the existence of each individual. The literature supports the view that many aspects of hope are not necessarily connected to cure but despite this there remains empirical evidence that health professionals still associate hope with cure or lack of progression of disease. This is of particular relevance when considering people who are dying from end-organ failure, where the hope of cure is elusive. The ability to maintain hope is enhanced by

(1) effective relief from distressing symptoms;
(2) the positive presence of a team of professional staff who can provide meaningful relationships with the patient;
(3) the perceived existence of a positive future for the patient and their family;
(4) the patient's feeling that they are valued as a person;
(5) the redefinition of the patient's goals as they move through the disease process.

A significant threat to maintaining hope is the individual's loss of control that threatens the existence of any future. Many social and psychological interventions are therefore well suited to a more positive view of hope in people with non-malignant disease.

In a review of health professionals' responses to MS and MND, Carter *et al.* 1998 found a small body of literature that examined aspects of health professionals' responses to neuromuscular disorders such as MS and MND. They confirmed from their own work that health professionals often find it difficult to maintain hope in the face of progressive neuromuscular diseases. They identified a number of reasons why they were able to convey hope. These included setting short-term goals and focusing on positive events; the effectiveness of certain interventions, for example, specific equipment, special techniques, or treatments for improving quality of life; and their dependence on the coping ability or outlook of the patients. When looking at not conveying hope the reasons included such items as the inevitable downward progression; the incurable nature of the disorder; the increasing disability of the patient; and strong identification with the patients or their families. Whilst the study found differences between responses to MS and MND, the authors drew conclusions about suggested ways in which the maintenance of hope may be enhanced, including such items as improving communication and liaison between health professionals in different settings, the development of a coordinated approach to service delivery, and the increased ability to set short-term goals and to develop new strategies for framing hope.

The maintenance of quality of life

The maintenance of quality of life remains a key component of palliative care whether the patient has a malignant or non-malignant disease. Quality-of-life measures that have largely been developed by clinicians and academics were initially used to measure group outcomes related to quality of care, the need for care, and the effectiveness of healthcare interventions (Carr and Higginson 2001). The lack of agreement in the definition of quality of life means that many of the measures do not have any underlying theoretical conceptualization, which means it is difficult to know what phenomena they are in fact measuring. Many tools have however been developed and features of these tools include that

(1) they are standardized measures containing preselected domains;

(2) they are uni-dimensional;

(3) the quality of life is expressed in quantifiable terms such as scores.

The usefulness of quality of life as an outcome may be limited because of a number of factors including

(1) lack of agreement in the definition of quality of life;

(2) lack of relevance of expert-derived measures to patients;

(3) debate about who is most appropriate to measure quality of life;

(4) problems inherent in quality-of-life measurement;

(5) limitations in the uni-dimensional structure of the tools.

An interactive model of 'living with dying' has been developed (MacLeod *et al.* in press) emphasizing the interconnectedness of themes rather than considering them as separate entities. The themes that were identified are personal and intrinsic factors, external and extrinsic factors, future issues, perceptions of normality, and taking charge. This latter component of taking charge proved to be an overarching element that assumed that people who were dying play a more active role in 'control'. This involved recognizing and actualizing their needs by either assuming total control or delegating some or all of it. The notion of taking charge appears to overlap with the concept of self-governance as described by Chochinov *et al.* (2002) but its scope is wider in that it is not restricted to matters relating to death but rather encompasses a range of matters concerned with both life and death. It is the patient's experience of how much control they perceive they have that is pivotal to their perceptions of well-ness, self-esteem, and hopefulness. Taking charge can be articulated by the active relinquishing of control (McKinlay 2001) and relinquishing control may enable people to focus on other domains such as interpersonal relationships, involvement in life, and a redefinition of normality where life now is compared to life without disease.

The maintenance of dignity

In their study on dignity in the terminally ill, Chochinov *et al.*, whilst undertaking work with people with advanced cancer, have identified major dignitary categories, themes, and sub-themes which are possibly transferable to people with non-malignant disease (Chochinov *et al.* 2002). The three main categories are

(1) illness-related concerns—these relate to the level of independence (cognitive acuity and functional capacity) and the level of symptom distress (both physical and psychological);

(2) dignity-conserving repertoire—this includes dignity-conserving perspectives (such as the continuity of self, role preservation, and the maintenance of pride, hopefulness, autonomy and control, and acceptance and resilience) and dignity-conserving practices (such as living in the moment, maintaining normalcy, and seeking spiritual comfort);

(3) social dignity inventory—this identifies sub-themes such as privacy boundaries, social support, the concept of being a burden to others, and concerns about the aftermath of their dying, along with the attitudes to caring of those around them.

Dignity therefore takes a key position in the maintenance of well-being in people approaching the end of life whether or not they have a malignant disease. Loss of dignity may enhance depression, hopelessness, and a desire for hastened death so it is essential that continued work is undertaken to pursue an understanding of dignity in people dying from non-malignant disease.

The maintenance of creativity

Music and art therapy can be useful adjuncts in the management of non-malignant disease, as they are with malignant disease, and they often have an impact on psychological or social well-being. In this context, music therapy is the controlled use of music, its elements, and their influences on the human being to aid in the physiological, psychological, and emotional integration of the individual during an illness.

By mobilizing deeply held beliefs and feelings it can assist in communication. From a psychological point of view it can help in identifying and reinforcing self-concept and self-worth, it can help to improve the patient's mood, it can help with recall of past significant events, and it can help in exploring fantasy and imagery. From a social point of view it can act as a means of socially acceptable self-expression, recreating a bond and a sense of community with family members, as a link to the patient's life before illness, and as entertainment and diversion. Restoring creativity to the dying patient has long been held as an important goal of palliative care teams. As with music therapy, art can be used to help to promote a healthy and safe environment. For the purposes of definition, art can include all forms of creative and interpretative expression. Other aspects of the arts, which have been used successfully in the management of symptoms near the end of life, include biography work, journalling, reminiscence therapy, and poetry. It has been suggested that we can express in written words things that we find hard to say and so poetry and prose can have a significant part to play in the discovery of the journey towards the end of life. The arts can also provide a most effective means by which a legacy can be left for the family. During the preparation of such items, a focus on relieving symptoms such as breathlessness can be maintained (MacLeod in press).

The future

Kellehear (1999) has argued powerfully that among the underdeveloped areas of palliative care are the social science and public health perspectives as well as the social side of care. His belief is that health promoting palliative care should be about providing education and information for health, dying, and death. It should provide social supports, especially personal and community supports, and it should also encourage interpersonal problem solving where this is relevant. The encouragement of a re-orientation of traditional palliative care services in order that we combat death denying health policies and attitudes in the wider society is needed. This will include a greater emphasis in the multi-disciplinary approach on those more skilled at psychological and social interventions for people dying from any disease.

One of the key tasks of educators is to ensure that a broader approach to learning to care for people who are dying is encompassed than is currently widely practised. At undergraduate level this means embracing a wider view of care than is generally adopted. In many countries most medical and nursing schools offer some formal training in end-of-life care, albeit predominantly care for people with malignant disease. This teaching is often viewed favourably by students, positively influences their attitudes, and enhances communication skills (Billings and Block 1997). There are however calls for a more systematic approach than is currently available (Emanuel 1997). The lack of adequate conceptualization of all palliative care, the significance of psychological, emotional, and spiritual aspects of care, its multi-professional nature, and the fact that caregivers have to perform their duties in situations where the psychological and emotional demands on them may be immense, are among items that have been seen to be problematic in education in palliative care (James and MacLeod 1993). There are developments that are encouraging though. A revision of basic core competencies for end-of-life care that includes psychological, sociological, and spiritual issues, interviewing and communication skills, management of common symptoms, ethical issues, and self-knowledge and self-reflection has been proposed (Barnard *et al.* 1999). Others have developed more experiential approaches to teaching (MacLeod and Robertson 1999) and more recently an interprofessional approach that identifies teamwork in the learning experience involving family carers to identify issues of significance for the students has been reported (Wee *et al.* 2001). This latter approach models teamwork by including skilled health and social care professionals as teachers along with the informal carers. Graduate and postgraduate work has shown that changes can be effected in more than the physical aspects of care. In a study of the effectiveness of a number of palliative care education programmes nurses identified changes in many of the psychosocial aspects of care to be a result of those courses (Kenny 2001). Similar changes are occurring in medical education (Fins and Nilson 2000; Sahler *et al.* 2000) with the development of a clearer understanding of what is particular about caring from a medical perspective.

The emphasis on the care of people with non-malignant disease will change as clinicians and teachers recognize the different facets of care needed to address the needs of people dying from those diseases. A re-focusing on aspects identified in this chapter will ensure that all health professionals caring for people at the end of life will be equipped to deal with a broad range of issues concerning not only death from malignant disease but also from the multiplicity of non-malignant diseases that are perhaps marginalized at present in education in this area.

References

Addington-Hall J, Falhoury W, McCarthy M (1998). Specialist palliative care in nonmalignant disease. *Palliative Med* **12:**417–27.

Barnard D, Quill T, Hafferty FW, Arnold R, Plumb J, Bulger R *et al.* (1999). Preparing the ground: contributions of preclinical years to medical education about care near the end of life. *Acad Med* **74:**499–505.

Billings JA, Block S (1997). Palliative care in undergraduate medical education. *JAMA* **278:**733–8.

Branch WT (2000). The ethics of caring and medical education. *Acad Med* **75:**127–32.

Carr AJ, Higginson IJ (2001). Are quality of life measures patient-centred? *BMJ* **322:**1357–60.

Carter H, McKenna C, MacLeod R, Green R (1998). Health professionals' responses to multiple sclerosis and motor neurone disease. *Palliative Med* **12:**383–94.

Chochinov H, Hack T, McClement S, Kristjanson L, Harlos M (2002). Dignity in the terminally ill: a developing empirical model. *Soc Sci Med* **54:**433–43.

Christakis N, Asch D (1993). Biases in how physicians choose to withdraw life support. *Lancet* **342:**642–6.

Department of Health (1987). *The undiscovered country.* Wellington: Government Printing Office.

Emanuel EJ (1997). Care for dying patients [editorial]. *Lancet* **349:**1714.

Field D (1998). Special not different: general practitioners' accounts of their care of dying people. *Soc Sci Med* **46:**1111–20.

Field MJ, Cassel C (ed.) (1997). *Approaching death: improving care at the end of life.* Washington DC: Institute of Medicine, National Academy Press.

Fins JF, Nilson EG (2000). An approach to educating residents about palliative care and clinical ethics. *Acad Med* **75:**662–5.

Fisher M (1995). Psychological needs and care in the hospice setting. *Eur J Palliative Care* **2:**115–19.

George R, Sykes J (1997). Beyond cancer? In: Clark D, Hockley J, Ahmedzai S (ed.). *New themes in palliative care.* Buckingham: Open University Press, p. 243.

Hall KH (2002). Reviewing intuitive decision-making and uncertainty: the implications for medical education. *Med Educ* **36:**216–24.

James CR, MacLeod RD (1993). The problematic nature of education in palliative care. *J Palliative Care* **9:**5–10.

Kashiwagi T (1995). Psychosocial and spiritual issues in terminal care. *Psychiat Clin Neurosci* **49 (suppl 1):**S123–127.

Katz J (1984). *The silent world of doctor and patient.* New York: Free Press.

Kellehear A (1999). *Health promoting palliative Care.* Australia: Oxford University Press.

Kenny LJ (2001). Education in palliative care: making a difference to practice? *Int J Palliative Nursing* **7:**401–7.

Kite S, Jones K, Tookman A (1999). Specialist palliative care and patients with noncancer diagnoses: the experience of a service. *Palliative Med* **13:**477–84.

Kleinman A (1988). *The illness narratives.* New York, USA: Basic Books.

Kutner JS, Steiner JF, Corbett KK, Jahnigen DW, Barton PL (1999). Information needs in terminal illness. *Soc Sci Med* **48:**1341–52.

McKinlay E (2001). Within the circle of care: patient experiences of receiving palliative care. *J Palliative Care* **17:**22–9.

MacLeod R (2000). Learning to care: a medical perspective. *Palliative Med* **14:**209–16.

MacLeod RD (in press) Dyspnoea—management: psychosocial therapies. In: Ahmedzai S, Muers M (ed.). *Oxford textbook—supportive care in respiratory disease.*

Macleod S (2001). Multiple sclerosis and palliative medicine. *Prog Palliative Care* **9:**196–8.

MacLeod R, Carter H (1999). Health professionals' perception of hope: understanding its significance in the care of people who are dying. *Mortality* **4:**309–17.

MacLeod RD, Robertson G (1999). Teaching and learning about living and dying: medical undergraduate palliative care education in Wellington, New Zealand. *Ed Health* **12:**185–92.

MacLeod R, Carter H, Brander P, McPherson K (in press). Living with a terminal illness.

McPherson KM, Brander P, McNaughton H, Taylor (2001). Living with arthritis—what is important? *Dis Rehab* **23:**706–21.

Massarotto A, Carter H, MacLeod R, Donaldson N (2000). Hospital referrals to a hospice: timing of referrals, referrers' expectations and the nature of referral information. *J Palliative Care* **16:**22–9.

National Council for Hospice and Specialist Palliative Care Services (1997). Feeling better: psychosocial care in specialist palliative care. London; April 1997. Occasional Paper No. 13.

Nursing Council (1996). Guidelines for cultural safety in nursing and midwifery education. Wellington: Nursing Council of New Zealand.

Oliviere D (1999). Culture and ethnicity *Eur J Palliative Care* **6:**53–6.

Oneschuk D (2001). Progressive multifocal leuko-encephalopathy and sporadic Creutzfeldt–Jacob disease: a review and palliative management in a hospice setting. *Prog Palliative Care* **9:**202–5.

Sahler OJ, Frager G, Levetown M, Cohn FG, Lipson MA (2000). Medical education about end-of-life care in the pediatric setting: principles, challenges and opportunities. *Pediatrics* **105:**575–84.

Seale C (1991). Death from cancer and death from other causes: the relevance of the hospice approach. *Palliative Med* **5:**12–19.

Steinke EE (1997). Sexuality in aging: implications for nursing facility staff. *J Cont Ed Nursing* **28:**59–63.

SUPPORT Principal Investigators (1996). A controlled trial to improve care for seriously ill hospitalized patients: The Study to Understand Prognoses and Preferences for Outcomes and Risks of Treatments (SUPPORT). *JAMA* **274:**1591–8.

Watson J (1988). Human care in nursing. In: Watson J (ed.). *Nursing: human science and human care. A theory of nursing.* New York: National League for Nursing Press. pp. 27–30.

Wee B, Hillier R, Coles C, Mountford B, Sheldon F, Turner P (2001). Palliative care: a suitable setting for undergraduate interprofessional education. *Palliative Med* **15:**487–92.

Chapter 9

Spiritual care

Mark Cobb

Introduction

We die because our bodies fail us. Weighed down by the burden of disease, physical trauma, or simply age, our life systems malfunction, our biology becomes disordered and we begin the inexorable journey towards death. This lethal sequence of events may be challenged through medical interventions but sooner or later the mortal nature of being human asserts its inevitable conclusion. However, this physical description of the end of life is an incomplete account of dying and an inadequate basis to provide care. A dying person is more than their pathology and patients want to be attended to as more than a terminal illness. Consequently, palliative care has committed itself to address the whole person through what have become conventionally referred to as the physical, psychological, social, and spiritual dimensions.

This chapter is concerned with the spiritual dimension and specifically how it applies to clinical practice. Spirituality as a concept is not without its problems and difficulties (Cobb 2001) but it has always had a place in the hospice movement and it continues to be a challenging presence in palliative care (Wright 2001). The term has strong religious roots in the Judaeo-Christian tradition and it can refer to a range of theological meanings and religious practices, not necessarily Jewish or Christian. It is also used in palliative care to refer to an intrinsic characteristic of an individual that can exist without necessary reference to a tradition or external body of beliefs. Spirituality is not therefore one thing and it may be helpful to regard it as category of phenomena that have individual and social manifestations. The spiritual dimension of palliative care is an attempt to recognize human experience that takes us beyond our immediate selves. Spirituality is therefore concerned with an aspect of human nature that is rooted in our experience of relatedness to both an inner and an outer world. For many this presents the possibility of a unique journey towards wholeness and which can be the source of meaning and growth even when life is drawing towards its end.

Spiritual issues towards the end of life

It's official, then. After nine months of talking bravely about 50:50 survival rates ... of bone disease being a really 'good' form of secondary breast cancer ... of a new, 'natural' chemotherapy regime which is showing really promising results ... of confident declarations of recovery from my healer and Chinese doctor ... I now have a brain tumour. Oh, and by the way, the lurgy is advancing rapidly into my liver and lungs, so there's no point in continuing with treatment. So no more false dawns, no more miracle cures, no more Alien-style eruptions of disease (I now have a 'full house' of secondary breast cancer sites—or 'mets', as we professionals like to say). The bottom line is, I'm dying. (Picardie 1998)

Beliefs

People take different stances towards death and this depends upon the way they make sense of their lives and the world view they inhabit, or to put it another way, their beliefs. In dialogue with culture, life history, and the way reality is conceived these beliefs provide a dependable framework of meaning within which people understand and respond to experiences and events. When this meaning extends beyond a materialistic account and includes a transcendent reality then we are dealing with matters of faith. The language of faith refers to that which is fundamentally important or real to people and transcendent reality is traditionally associated in the Western context with terms such as God, the Holy, and the Eternal. The major religious traditions have their own descriptions of ultimate reality (Hick 1999) and these provide the basis for beliefs around which people can pattern and direct their lives. However, for a person who does not hold to any particular faith tradition may still adopt a spiritual orientation and inhabit a world view that includes the transcendent. Spirituality is therefore not simply an intellectual proposition but consists of cognitive, emotional, and behavioural components (Argyle 2000) that contribute to defining the person and to the way life is experienced.

When people have to contemplate their own death, they have to contemplate the end of themselves and their non-existence in the world as they know it. A diagnosis of terminal illness signals that life is not inviolable and that the frail and fragile body through which we experience and live in the world will fail us. Mortality is a challenge to life and it is a challenge to the beliefs we hold about life. From the questions of 'Why me?' to those about life beyond death, beliefs will shape the way people respond to their ailing health and eventually to their death. People's experience of being ill and dying will also impact upon their beliefs and there may be contradictions that become evident between their beliefs and their experience. Some can hold these tensions whilst others may seek to resolve them but we are reminded of the dynamic nature of beliefs and the significance they can have for a person.

Spiritual beliefs can often come into focus at a time of transition and change. These beliefs may have been dormant or latent for many years, or they may be contemporary, but they can be invoked when someone is trying to make sense of disruptions to the life journey and in particular to a terminal condition. Spiritual beliefs can give meaning to experience but more practically they can provide the basis upon which patients respond to care, choose treatment options, and face their death. What may seem to be abstract spiritual beliefs are therefore situated in a personal context that exists in relationship to a wider social network of family, friends, and caregivers. Spiritual beliefs may be consistent both within this network and with the philosophy of a palliative care service. However, there may be abrasion or conflicts between differing beliefs that impinge directly on decisions affecting care and treatment (Hamel and Lysaught 1994). Issues concerning quality of life, the nature and meaning of pain, the need to fulfil end-of-life tasks, and accepting the finality of life may all throw into relief differences in belief that may require some resolution. Discrepancy in views, and particularly a negative or uncertain attitude, may signal to a patient a disinterest by clinicians or discrimination against such beliefs.

An important aspect of spiritual beliefs in palliative care is that they may contribute to the way in which a person copes with a terminal illness. In a study of patients with malignant melanoma, those who rated high religious and spiritual beliefs often used active–cognitive means of coping. The researchers suggested that beliefs may provide patients with a sense of connection, involvement, and meaning that helps them to accept their illness (Holland *et al.* 1999).

However, whilst for some people beliefs contribute to coping, for others they may be ineffective or even problematic. Stressful life events challenge a person's world view and they can put a strain on beliefs. Negative aspects of coping may result when there is a disintegration of beliefs evident in doubts, confusion, conflict, and distress. It should be noted that what may be interpreted as problematic to a clinician may to a patient be an opportunity to wrestle with beliefs and to reappraise them (Pargament *et al.* 1998). What this suggests is that learning what it means to be dying may involve spiritual growth and enrichment.

Faith practices and rituals

Spirituality for many people is not simply a concept or category but has practical, social, and material expressions and manifestations. The practical aspects of spirituality may involve activities such as rituals, prayer, meditation, sacramental rites, and pilgrimage. Spirituality also exists in social forms, most notably through religious traditions, institutions, and functionaries, but it can also be found expressed in group values, beliefs, and morals. Spirituality is therefore embodied in people's lives and actions as well as in concrete material forms (Smart 1996). Chapels, temples, mosques, icons, rosaries, holy books, and symbols can all be considered material expressions of the spiritual. It is therefore important when approaching spiritual issues that form as well as content are considered and explored.

Patients come into contact with palliative care service because of their diagnosis and not because of their faith or beliefs. Patients may have practices and rituals that they wish to maintain and observe because of their faith and beliefs. Illness and its consequences can interfere with the routines of life and the habits through which people sustain meaning. Faith practices can be interrupted by healthcare commitments and patients can be easily dislocated from their faith communities and the people who support them in their religious beliefs and customs. In particular people from minority faith traditions may find it difficult to access the support they need (Gilliat-Ray 2001). For patients who currently have no connection to a faith community the obligations of being a patient or the limitations of illness can restrict the possibilities they have of wanting to return to a former community or of making new connections.

People who observe faith practices, rituals, festivals, and ceremonies do so for a range of reasons but they may find them affirming and sustaining, particularly in the face of change and uncertainty. Faith practices may help to maintain a sense of personal identity as well as connectedness to a faith community. For this reason beliefs and practices cannot be separated from the social dynamic of culture. Faith practices are not generic and ignorance, stereotyped assumptions, or the rigid categorization of practices can obscure the actual needs of individuals. When a patient has a clearly identified religious faith then specific practices may be identified. However, people of nominal or no expressed religious commitment may still employ faith practices, such as prayer or meditation, or wish to participate in religious ritual.

Finally in considering rituals and faith practices in the context of palliative care we have to take account of those that concern the dead. Rituals around death underscore the transition from life to death and help people to let go. Rituals following death serve a very functional purpose of last offices and the disposal of the corpse but they also provide a framework of meaning, beliefs, and behaviour that can enable the bereaved to make sense of their loss (Davies 1997). There may therefore be a span of ritual practice that begins when a person is approaching death and continues through to acts of remembrance and memorialization. The faith traditions provide a rich source of ritual practice that people can draw upon but those who have no connection with a faith community may still seek ritual expression for their grief.

Suffering

Terminal illness is an assault on the integrity of the person and suffering can result in a variety of ways. In addition to the bodily burdens resulting from symptoms of the disease a patient can suffer through the many dimensions of personhood. This is because a terminal illness is a threat to a person's existence in the world and to life's goals. These include social roles and identity, relatedness to self and others, well-being, and fulfilment. People can suffer therefore when the integrity of their personhood is damaged or as a result of some form of irrecoverable loss. When people cannot make sense of what is happening to them, and particularly when they can find no place for it within their framework of meaning, then suffering may be related to the spiritual dimension (Van Hooft 1998).

Suffering is not the result of a simple cause-and-effect mechanism, it is always particular to the person and it is temporal. People may accept suffering and leave it unchallenged but many find a resilience to respond to suffering. This enforced challenge may constitute striving for a new sense of wholeness and the self that emerges through biographical work in which the illness is incorporated or transcended. Transcendence enables connectedness and removes the isolation of suffering by setting it within a 'larger landscape' and through bringing people close to sources of ultimate meaning (Cassel 1982). The religious traditions of the world have their own interpretations of suffering and many have practices that enable people to transcend their immediate selves through prayer, meditation, and ritual. Whilst they acknowledge the reality of suffering, they point towards an ultimate goodness of the universe and the fulfilment of the human soul beyond suffering.

Suffering, however, may be unfathomable for people, it may persist and it can overwhelm. In these circumstance people speak of injustice, hopelessness, darkness, and despair. Any faith a patient may have had can appear shattered, they can feel abandoned, and hell can seem a very present reality. Spiritual suffering can be related at this level to depression and a psychiatric assessment may help in determining whether the patient has a mood disorder that may benefit from treatment or if the patient is at risk of suicide. This degree of suffering can be difficult to endure for carers and there are no quick remedies to lighten the troubled spirit. Patients may literally give up, become withdrawn, and become disconnected from people. The spiritual challenge for carers is to be able to contain this sense of dereliction and maintain a consistent presence that may bear witness to the possibility of connectedness once again.

Death

It can be difficult to grasp the fact of death from a personal perspective and people with a terminal illness may avoid anticipating the end of their lives. But for those who do contemplate it, there can be significant spiritual issues arising from what results from this fatal event. Some people hold that the result of death is simply nothing, or to be more accurate the permanent absence of the dead person from the world with its resultant losses for the bereaved. Many people with a religious commitment place death within the transcendent possibilities of the eternal and attempt to live their life in preparation for this reality. But what all these accounts have in common is the question of human destiny and it is this that patients, out of self-interest alone, may wish to explore.

In a detailed study of the last months of nine terminally ill people, researchers reported that participants, regardless of their spiritual or religious orientation, searched for 'some tangible evidence of continuity with ongoing life after their own death' (Staton *et al.* 2001). Transcending physical death for these people was in part about finding a connection with something that endured and this seemed to be related to accepting the finality of their existence. This was expressed both through a notion of a tangible legacy, such as passing on valued objects or property, and an intangible spiritual connection with others, creation, and the transcendent. Death can therefore be seen as something of a spiritual boundary that marks both the cessation of life and a re-integration of the self with the natural world or the infinite.

Exploring what death means to people can often betray their deepest fears and hopes; paradoxically the anticipation of decay and death can also hold the expectation of liberation. Symbolic images and stories are often the means for contemplating death and many can be found in the religious traditions. However, contemporary culture also supplies plentiful examples that express ideas of death and destiny through fiction, songs, and films. Here we may find a mixture of Western and Eastern thought in which eternal life in heaven coexists with reincarnation or rebirth in this world. These attempts to make sense of death and find meaning in it can provide the starting point for a patient and here the creative arts can provide a language and means of personal exploration. But however it is engaged with by patients it also needs to be engaged with by carers. As with other spiritual aspects of palliative care this may prove

to be challenging and difficult but without this consideration staff may unintention-
ally obstruct attempts by patients to contemplate death and therefore prevent them
from engaging with a meaningful part of their dying.

Providing spiritual care

The philosophy of palliative care is premised on an understanding of personhood that
includes the spiritual dimension. But what does this mean for the actual practice of
care and the delivery of services? Can we understand spiritual care in the same way as
other types of care and how can it be resourced and organized? If spiritual care is to
be translated from an abstract philosophical concept into the practice of palliative care
then we need some clarity about what it involves and the framework within which it
operates. As we have already discussed, spirituality is not one thing and it may be
understood as a category of phenomena with individual and social manifestations.
This broad approach allows for a wide spectrum of spiritual orientations from those
that can be highly differentiated as religious to those that have no reference to faith
traditions and are markedly humanistic and personal. The benefit of this approach is
that it is an attempt at being inclusive of the range of spiritualities that are found
among patients. This should not be a fudge of the very real differences that exist
between different spiritual orientations, nor an attempt at reaching the lowest
common denominator, but a means of accommodating the breadth of spirituality that
people present.

The variety of spiritual beliefs, experiences, and practices that coexist in the population served will be depend on demographic, cultural, and social factors. Religion will
constitute an obvious part of the spiritual terrain and socially and culturally significant forms of religious life will be evident in organizations, worship places, and the
office holders of the faith communities (Weller 2000). However, whilst people may
associate themselves with religious beliefs they may not belong actively to a faith community or they may only turn to it when faced with major life events (Davie 1994).
Most healthcare services make some attempt to record the 'religion' of a patient but
beyond this cursory question there may be no further steps taken to enquire of the
patient's spirituality. Results from ongoing studies of the Royal Free interview for religious and spiritual beliefs suggest that spiritual issues may be more prevalent than
professionals sometimes accept and that 'patients are concerned with these aspects of
human experience and are able to express them if approached in an appropriate way'.
In a study of patients admitted to three acute wards, 175 of the 300 people who participated reported a religious and a spiritual belief, 32 a spiritual and not religious belief,
and 29 a philosophical belief. A later study reported that 80 per cent of cardiology
patients and 78 per cent of gynaecology patients who took part professed some form of
spiritual belief whether or not they engaged in religious activity (King et al. 1994).

There are some patients who will disclose their spirituality directly to healthcare professionals or indirectly through their faith practices, rituals, and symbols. Many will not
and professionals may lack the interest, confidence, understanding, or skills to explore
this area or identify concerns. Patients may also withhold their concerns in order to
appear that they are coping or if they perceive staff would not cope (Heaven and

Maguire 1997). The spiritual domain is one that can be subject to prejudice, presumption, and neglect and consequently patients may feel isolated and unsupported. What this suggests is that a consistent approach should be taken by palliative care services to ensure patients are given the opportunity to express their spiritual beliefs and practices. This will enable a service to acknowledge and respect the spiritual aspects of a patient and inform the provision of relevant support.

Assessment

If an assessment of a patient's spirituality is to be undertaken it cannot be simply out of the self-interest of the healthcare professional but because we think we can respond in some useful, caring, or supportive way. This is an important ethical dimension to assessment and one that needs to be considered carefully, given the strong reliance on a trustworthy relationship through which spirituality can be articulated. In addition, if an assessment is to be reliable and sensitive it must be informed, responsive to the particular patient, and mindful of the potential for the subject area to be problematic. Assessments in palliative care typically focus on pathology, problematic symptoms, and disruptions to well-being. Spirituality suffering can manifest itself through threats to personhood but there are also aspects of spirituality that would not be elicited in the search for problems because they are well integrated, positive, and fulfilling. The assessment therefore needs to incorporate this wider compass in order to capture as accurately as possible the patient's understanding of their spirituality. However, as one of the early writers on spiritual assessment noted

> the values and beliefs elicited in these areas may or may not be expressed by the person through conventional religious language and rituals. Some people may find these content areas vague, verbally incongruent with their behaviour, or even threatening to discuss. It is important, therefore, to acknowledge each person's right to his own values and beliefs and to respect his right to remain silent about them. (Stoll 1979)

Proceeding with these caveats and cautions it is important that a palliative care service has a properly considered and planned approach to assessing spirituality, and this raises a number of questions.

1. Which members of the team should initiate the assessment?
2. Is the assessment practicable for the sort of patients using the service?
3. Is it socially and culturally relevant to all or particular patients?
4. Are the language and concepts appropriate and congruent with the patient's?
5. Is the assessment responsive to the patient and able to cope with different levels of response?
6. Is the person carrying out the assessment competent to deal with the patient's responses and are there effective referral mechanisms in place?
7. Is the assessment process ongoing, comprehensive, and incorporated into care planning?
8. Is the assessment process consistent throughout the service?

The assessment process must begin by addressing the question of whether or not spirituality is important to a patient. Even this most basic stage in the process cannot proceed without good communication skills and an informed approach. Consideration must be given to the wording of questions and what may be known already about the patient (see Table 9.1). The patient's previous notes may contain data about religious affiliation and this may provide a starting point, 'I see from your notes that you describe your religion as Jewish, can you tell me about this?' If there are no data prior to meeting the patient then a broader and more open-ended type of question needs to be used, 'Do you have any spiritual or religious beliefs?' These questions are the first stage of the assessment process and should demonstrate to the patient that spirituality is respected and taken as seriously as other aspects of patient care.

Providing that the patient has indicated that this is a meaningful aspect of their life and that they are willing to talk about it, the assessment can move onto eliciting some outline description of the nature and significance of the patient's spirituality. Spirituality may have obvious form and content, or it may be more abstract, in which case the professional carrying out the assessment must ensure that the patient's description has been correctly understood and where there is doubt, clarification sought. Patients are often more than willing to explain the nature of their spirituality and what it means to them and it is one way for professionals to demonstrate their concern and respect.

Once an outline of a patient's spiritual orientation has been gained the next stage in the assessment is to ascertain how important and helpful it is. A simple question is often sufficient, 'Is your faith/spirituality/religion helpful to you?' or 'How important would you say this is to you?'. Patients may indicate that whilst they hold certain beliefs they are not something, at this time, which concerns them and the assessment can be

Table 9.1 Examples of helpful questions in an initial assessment

1	'I see from your notes that you describe your religion as Jewish, can you tell me about this?' *or if no data is available* 'Do you have any spiritual or religious beliefs?' 'Can you tell me about them?'
2	'Is your faith/spirituality/religion helpful to you?' *or* 'How important would you say this is to you?'
3	'Are they ways in which we can support you in your faith/spirituality/religion?' *or* 'Can we help provide you with anything or any facilities to support you in your faith/spirituality/religion?' 'Are there things we need to know about your faith/spirituality/religion that would help us in caring for you?'
4	'Would you like to talk with someone about these matters?' *or* 'We have a chaplain who is part of the team, would you like see them?' *or* 'Would you like us to arrange a member of your faith community to visit you?'

concluded with reassurance that if the patient wants to talk about their spirituality a member of the team will be happy to do so. If a patient indicates that their spiritual orientation is significant then the assessment needs to continue to establish how the patient may be supported in this. Questions can be open, 'Are they ways in which we can support you in your faith/spirituality/religion?' and practical, 'Can we help provide you with anything or any facilities to support you in your faith/spirituality/ religion?'. Equally it is important for a palliative care service to know about aspects of a patient's spiritual orientation that may promote or prohibit certain practices or that may be an important reference point in decision making, 'Are there things we need to know about your faith/spirituality/religion that would help us in caring for you?'.

Finally in an initial form of assessment the patient should be given the opportunity to speak further with someone, 'Would you like to talk with someone about these matters?' or 'We have a chaplain who is part of the team, would you like see them?'. It may be, depending upon previous answers, that the patient is already involved with a faith community and the more appropriate question might be, 'Would you like us to arrange a member of your faith community to visit you?' (Highfield 2000; Lo et al. 1999; Hodge 2001). This patient-led interview provides an assessment process that can be sensitive to the responses of patients but a more objective and systematic approach may be gained by using some form of patient-completed questionnaire (King et al. 2001).

An initial assessment provides basic information to enable a palliative care team to support a patient's spiritual orientation and to ensure the care plan is consistent with a patient's beliefs and practices. It should be recognized that an assessment interview may be therapeutically beneficent for a patient, in part because of the cathartic opportunity that it may present someone. As with other forms of assessment it is not a single event but needs to be an ongoing process. Professionals should be alert to the patient who has initially declined any discussion of spirituality but who may seek some form of spiritual care in the future. Spiritual assessment may also develop from more empirical or objective aspects into the subjective aspects of spirituality that require a more in-depth and attentive approach. The assessment process may therefore extend to more biographical and temporal aspects of spirituality (Hays et al. 2001; Speck 1998). Any form of assessment needs to be incorporated into care planning and it must be properly documented. Information gained about a patient's spiritual beliefs and practices should be evaluated alongside other aspects of the person within the multi-disciplinary team and be used to inform decisions about care and interventions. For example, a patient who would usually read the Bible, may, because of their illness need someone to read to them.

Modes of spiritual care

The form and type of spiritual care is best determined by the patient in consultation with a member of the professional team. There will be patients who will have their spiritual care needs met by people from their own faith community or others external to the team. In this case supportive arrangements need to be put in place to allow access and provide necessary facilities. For patients who are not involved with or do not wish to be referred to any external agency or for those with access difficulties, the

Table 9.2 Parameters of pastoral care

Pastoral care involves the establishment of a relationship or relationships whose purpose may encompass support in a time of trouble and personal or spiritual growth through deeper understanding of oneself, others, and/or God. Pastoral care will have at its heart the affirmation of meaning and worth of persons and will endeavour to strengthen their ability to respond creatively to whatever life brings.

To name such care as 'pastoral' is to locate it within a community of faith, either because of its setting or because the carer is a designated representative of that community.

Pastoral care is sensitive to the uniqueness of the spiritual journey of each human being, respecting the autonomy of individuals and their freedom to make their own choices.

Pastoral care enjoys a freedom, but not a compulsion, to draw upon the traditional resources of the community of faith, such as prayer, Scripture, and sacrament and the needs (stated or perceived) of the person receiving care being determinative.

team will need to facilitate spiritual care. As we have recognized throughout this chapter, spirituality is not one thing and therefore spiritual care is also a category covering different forms.

One of the principle modes of spiritual care is that of pastoral care. This primarily religious endeavour is theologically and psychologically informed and in its broadest sense is concerned with supporting people in times of need (Hunter 1990). Pastoral care operates within certain parameters, with reference to a faith tradition and is practised by a representative of a faith community (Table 9.2). This mode of spiritual care is most readily associated with the Judeo-Christian traditions and with the role of the healthcare chaplain but other faith traditions may also provide representatives with proximal roles (Lyall 2001).

Patients whose spirituality is not orientated around any particular faith tradition or is not related to any particular faith community may still benefit from a pastoral care approach. It will be important for both parties to have mutual respect and to maintain their own integrity. Beyond this mode spiritual care will operate within a more general psychological and therapeutic framework. This humanistic mode will be located in a patient's world view and their understanding. This is a supportive mode of spiritual care that aims at fostering positive coping and the enhancement of wellbeing. A humanistic approach to spiritual care will provide opportunities for patients to explore their spiritual beliefs and experience, to address concerns, and to empower them in their own spiritual journey. This mode will draw upon counselling skills and the relational context but it is not just problem focused and will involve sustaining positive aspects of spirituality.

Resources

The patient

It is not with the intention of objectifying the patient that we should consider them as a primary resource. It is in valuing the person's spiritual history, beliefs, and experiences that the resources within someone may emerge and be encouraged to develop. A patient, for example, may have a developed daily habit of prayer that seems difficult to sustain in an in-patient unit. Without regular prayer the patient may feel spiritually isolated and alone. Prayer requires attention and focus and with appropriate support, encouragement, and some practical rearrangements, the patient may be enabled to draw upon this deeply personal and transcendent aspect of their spirituality.

The patient's own resources may include spiritual practices and beliefs and they may involve significant people. It may be helpful for palliative care teams to have in mind some form of spiritual genogram for those patients whose spirituality has transpersonal and social aspects. The involvement of other people may be correspond to significant personal relationships, such as those of a partner or family, it may relate to people who have died but are still active in the person's worldview; or it may involve members of a faith community. This will need to be carefully and sensitively explored with the patient and could form part of an ongoing assessment.

The palliative care team

Who is responsible for providing spiritual care is a useful question for a team to discuss and respond to. Probably the only person with a specified responsibility will be that of the chaplain but many team members have an expectation of being able to provide some form of spiritual care. Nurses in particular consider this to be an aspect of their role. In a study of nurses almost half of them responded that they provided spiritual help and support for the terminally ill primarily by taking them to spiritual events on the ward, facilitating participation in Holy Communion, entering discussions about the meaning of life and God, and consulting with a chaplain. However, almost half of the nurses felt they had poor skills and knowledge in this area and over a third of the nurses were not willing to provide spiritual support (Kuuppelomäki 2001).

If a team is functioning well then it will appreciate the complementary skills and knowledge of its members. A chaplain who is properly integrated into a team should be an important resource to a team not only for direct patient care but also for advice and consultation. As part of the care planning a decision should be taken with the patient on who should be the lead person in facilitating and providing spiritual care. In this way spiritual care does not dissolve into some generic but marginal team function, nor does it exclude other members of the team from contributing.

Facilities

Palliative care services are hostages to architecture, competing demands on space, and financial restraints. The facilities originally planned for a service may no longer meet the current needs of service users and new or additional facilities may be required. For community-based services, access may be a real problem. Copies of sacred texts, prayer mats, and rosaries are all examples of small-scale equipment that may be easily obtained but more permanent facilities, such as prayer rooms, require long-term planning and financial commitment. In developing facilities, user involvement can ensure that what seems like a good idea 'on paper' is in reality useful and fulfils its intended purpose. In addition to specific facilities, spiritual care needs should be considered in all aspects of how a service operates and functions.

Faith communities

Local communities are important resources and should be involved in public services. In matters of spiritual care there is much that can be learnt from local faith communities and services need to develop effective mechanisms to allow this to happen. People are often very willing to be involved and it is important that hard-to-reach or minority groups are encouraged and supported in this. The involvement of faith communities may be strengthened by establishing a 'faith forum' to be involved in service developments and in providing relevant advice. The faith forum may also be an effective route through which to establish associate chaplains from minority faith groups.

Education, training, and professional development

Spirituality is a complex domain and one that requires different levels of skill, knowledge, and practice. If spirituality is an important dimension of palliative care then training programmes should be provided to resource staff with an adequate knowledge base and clinical skills. At present there are wide variations among disciplines and organizations as to what is available and a more systematic approach would be to include spiritual care within the educational strategy of a service (Johnson 1998). Spiritual care also requires more than the application of theory or knowledge because spirituality is necessarily a reflective and contemplative process. Professionals who work in this domain need to be resourced with some form of supervision in order to explore the impact of intimate personal encounters upon their own spirituality; to develop skills, and to face their own doubts, distress, prejudices, and defences (Hawking and Shohet 2000).

Conclusion

If we are to treat patients as whole people then spiritual care will not be something extraneous to palliative care. If we are to listen to patients and pay attention to their spiritual beliefs, experiences, and practices then professionals have a responsibility to integrate spiritual care into clinical practice. This can be a challenging aspect of care but it is one that can reveal the inspiring nature of the human spirit even in the face of death. Throughout this chapter we have been reminded that spirituality is not one thing and therefore spiritual care will be diverse. But whatever form it takes, spiritual care must be purposeful, properly resourced, and undertaken within a clear ethical framework. Inevitably professionals who develop skills and knowledge in this domain will need to address their own spirituality and mortality. In doing so they may deepen their own humanity and be more able to respond to the spiritual depths of others.

References

Argyle M (2000). *Psychology and religion.* London: Routledge.

Cassel EJ (1982). The nature of suffering and the goals of medicine. *New Engl J Med* **306:**639–45.

Cobb M (2001). *The dying soul: spiritual care at the end of life.* Buckingham: Open University Press.

Davie G (1994). *Religion in Britain since 1945.* Oxford: Blackwell.

Davies DJ (1997). *Death, ritual and belief.* London: Cassell.

Gilliat-Ray S (2001). Sociological perspective on the pastoral care of minority faiths in hospital. In: Orchard H (ed.). *Spirituality in health care contexts.* London: Jessica Kingsley.

Hamel RP, Lysaught MT (1994). Choosing palliative care: do religious beliefs make a difference? *J Palliative Care* **10:**61–6.

Hawking P, Shohet R (2000). *Supervision in the helping professions.* Buckingham: Open University Press.

Hays JC, Meador KG, Branch PS, George LK (2001). The spiritual history scale in four dimensions (SHS-4): validity and reliability. *Gerontologist* **41:**239–49.

Heaven CM, Maguire P (1997). Disclosure of concerns by hospice patients and their identification by nurses. *Palliative Med* **11:**283–90.

Hick J (1999). *The fifth dimension: an exploration of the spiritual realm.* Oxford: Oneworld.

Highfield MEF (2000). Providing spiritual care to patients with cancer. *Clin J Oncol Nursing* **4:**115–20.

Hodge DR (2001). Spiritual assessment: a review of major qualitative methods and a new framework for assessing spirituality. *Soc Work* **46:**203–14.

Holland JC, Passik S, Kash KM, Russak S, Gronert M, Sison A *et al.* (1999). The role of religious and spiritual beliefs in coping with malignant melanoma. *Pscho-oncology* **8:**14–26.

Hunter RJ (1990). *Dictionary of pastoral care and counselling.* Nashville: Abingdon.

Johnson A (1998). The notion of spiritual care in professional practice. In: Cobb M, Robshaw V (ed.). *The spiritual challenge of health care.* Edinburgh: Churchill Livingstone.

King M, Speck P, Thomas A (1994). Spiritual and religious beliefs in acute illness—is this a feasible area for study? *Soc Sci Med* **38:**636.

King M, Speck P, Thomas A (2001). The Royal Free interview for spiritual and religious beliefs: development and validation of a self-report version. *Psychol Med* **31:**1015–23.

Kuuppelomäki M (2001). Spiritual support for terminally ill patients: nursing staff assessments. *J Clin Nursing* **20:**660–70.

Lo B, Quill T, Tulsky J (1999). Discussing palliative care with patients. *Ann Intern Med* **130:**744–9.

Lyall D (2001). *Integrity of pastoral care.* London: Society for the Propagation of Christian Knowledge.

Pargament KI, Zinnbauer BJ, Scott AB, Butter EM, Zerowin J, Stanik P (1998). Red flags and religious coping: identifying some religious warning signs among people in crisis. *J Clin Psychol* **54:**77–89.

Picardie R (1998). *Before I say goodbye.* London: Penguin.

Smart N (1996). *Dimensions of the sacred.* London: Harper Collins.

Speck P (1998). Spiritual issues in palliative care. In: Doyle D, Hanks GWC, MacDonald N (ed.). *Oxford textbook of palliative medicine.* Oxford: Oxford University Press.

Staton J, Shuy R, Byock I (2001). *A few months to live: different paths to life's end.* Washington DC: Georgetown University Press.

Stoll RI (1979). Guidelines for spiritual assessment. *Am J Nursing* **9:**1574–7.

Van Hooft S (1998). Suffering and the goals of medicine. *Med Health Care Philos* **1:**125–31.

Weller P (2000). *Religions in the UK: directory 2001–2003.* Derby: University of Derby.

Wright MC (2001). Spirituality: a developing concept within palliative care? *Prog Palliative Care* **9:**143–8.

Chapter 10

Bereavement care

Sheila Payne and Mari Lloyd-Williams

Introduction

Academics, poets, and novelists have written many words about bereavement and loss but in everyday life our most common experience is being at a 'loss for words' when these momentous events happen (Plate 4, pp. 98–99). The feeling of not being able to explain and describe our grief is common in the immediate aftermath of a death. Also many of us are at a loss to know what to say to those who are recently bereaved. Health professionals may worry about saying the 'wrong' thing or trying to find the 'right' words to comfort bereaved relatives. Finding the words to offer support is perhaps even more difficult if the bereaved person is a child. This chapter is about the language and discourses of bereavement. We will trace the ways of talking and understanding bereavement back to some of the theoretical ideas that emerged in the last century. Some ways of talking and thinking about bereavement have become so popular that many people are unaware of their origins and they have become part of our taken-for-granted knowledge about bereavement.

It is generally agreed that there are no single 'correct' or 'true' theories that explain the experience of loss or account for the emotions, experiences, and cultural practices which characterize grief and mourning (Payne *et al.* 1999; Hockey *et al.* 2001). A postmodern position suggests that individual diversity is paramount and that within broad cultural constraints each of us develops our own ways of 'doing' bereavement (Walter 1999). This accords well with many health professionals' experiences and awareness of the range of responses from their patients and clients. Although there may not appear to be strict social rules on how to behave when bereaved in this country, Hockey (2001) has highlighted that there are more subtle injunctions 'that the individual shall express their emotions, shall acknowledge the reality of their loss and shall share their thoughts and feelings with appropriate others'. Many bereavement support services operate with these basic requirements of their clients.

This chapter explores how dominant theories of loss have shaped our understanding of bereavement. We offer a brief introduction to psychiatric and psychological theories, followed by more recent models derived from theories of stress and coping. Latterly, theories have emphasized continuity and integration and we will review their implications. Whilst we will endeavour to draw on theories and research, which extend understanding of loss beyond Western cultural norms, much of this chapter is grounded in our research and practice in the UK. We are aware of much diversity but cannot adequately reflect this in one short chapter. The chapter will show how theoretical ideas have been incorporated into notions of 'normal' bereavement and the roles health professionals play in facilitating what most regard as a 'process'. We will draw on research that has examined how general practitioners and primary care-based counsellors talk about bereavement and their work with clients. Most hospices and palliative care services regard the provision of bereavement support as integral to their services. Yet there has been great diversity in how these services are organized and delivered. We will argue that this has been one of the most marginalized aspects of hospice development and will try to identify the reasons for this (Payne 2001a). The chapter concludes with a discussion about childhood bereavement services.

Theories of grief and bereavement

Most cultures have ideas about what happens after death and how bereaved people should feel and behave. Historical and archaeological evidence provide plenty of examples, perhaps the best known being ancient Egyptian tombs with their embalmed bodies and memorials. In our own times the range of beliefs, practices, and rituals associated with death and mourning is impressively large (see Parkes *et al.* 1997). Most religions provide accounts for what happens after death and may prescribe predeath thoughts and behaviours such as the 'last rites' given by Roman Catholic priests or the mouthful of Ganges water for dying Hindus (Firth 2001). Most major religions also provide guidance on how bereaved people should respond after the death, although these behaviours and practices may be modified over time due to changes such as migration. For example, Firth (2001) describes how UK Hindus have had to adapt cremation and associated death rituals to the constraints of UK crematoria. It is important to acknowledge that ideas derived from religious teaching have evolved and continue to do so. However, the UK has become an increasingly secular society and arguably, religious teaching provides less guidance than in the past.

It is appropriate at this point to consider the meaning of the terms that we will use in this chapter. The common root of the words bereavement and grief (reave) is derived from the Old English word 'reafian', to plunder, spoil, or rob (Oxford English Dictionary 1989). Two aspects of loss by death—the sense of personal violation and the heaviness of the soul—are thus embedded in the language itself (Payne *et al.* 1999). Bereavement is usually considered to be the process surrounding the loss of a loved object. In the context of this chapter, this is a person who has died, but it may also refer to loss of significant relationships, a way of life, a pet, a belief, or anything that has personal meaning for the individual. The reaction to this loss is grief. There is much debate as to whether grief is a universal human response to bereavement and loss. Mourning is generally described as the behavioural, emotional, and cognitive expression of grief. Mourning is heavily influenced by cultural and gender-specific norms. For example, in some cultures women do not attend funerals. While it appears simple and straightforward to separate out these aspects of loss into neat definitions,

Small (2001) has argued that they are intimately linked to our theoretical understanding of loss. So the language we use to describe bereavement both reveals and shapes our understanding of this experience.

Developmental theories

The first group of theories that will be discussed are based on developmental notions of change and growth. They make the assumption that bereavement is a 'process' in which there is an 'outcome'. The idea of process is typically expressed as phases, stages, or tasks to be accomplished. Notions of change and process are fundamental and failure to 'move on' or 'progress' gives rise to ideas of being 'stuck'. The theories have largely concentrated their attention on the intrapsychic domain, the inner workings of the mind. They have emphasized how people think and especially how they feel, their emotions. There is also an assumption that people have some control over their feelings and thoughts, and that these can be accessed through talk. Moreover, they suggest that successful grieving requires effortful mental processing called 'grief work' and that failure to do this is 'abnormal'. So where do these ideas come from?

The most influential and earliest theories of bereavement emerged from the psychoanalytic tradition, perhaps the most important being those of Freud (1917). Freud contributed much to twentieth century thought and his ideas have been very influential in shaping our ways of understanding people. In 1917, Freud first pointed out the similarities and differences between grief and depression in his classic text 'Mourning and melancholia'. His paper offered one of the first descriptions of normal and pathological grief. The thoughts discussed in it underpin psychoanalytic theory of depression and provide the base for many current theories of grief and its resolution. In the light of the impact of Freud's theory of grief on subsequent theoretical developments, it is surprising to acknowledge that grief, as a psychological process, was never Freud's main focus of interest. In the paper, he argued that people became attached to others who are important for the satisfaction of their needs and to whom emotional expression is directed. Love is conceptualized as the attachment of emotional energy to the psychological representation of the loved person. It is assumed that the more important the relationship, the greater the degree of attachment. According to Freudian theory, grieving represents a dilemma because there is a simultaneous need to relinquish the relationship so that the person may regain the energy invested and a wish to maintain the bond with the loved object. The individual needs to accept the reality of the loss so that the emotional energy can be released and redirected. The process of withdrawing energy from the lost object is called 'grief work'. He regarded this intrapsychic processing as essential to the breaking of relationship bonds with the deceased and to allow the reinvestment of emotional energy and the formation of new relationships with others. Arguably Freud's most important contributions to loss have been

(1) introducing a developmental perspective (his personality theory emphasized early childhood development);
(2) introducing the 'grief work' hypothesis;
(3) defining the difference between grief and depression.

His ideas were taken up and developed by many other people such as Lindemann (1944), Fenichel (1945) and Sullivan (1956). We will just mention a few important theorists. In the second half of the twentieth century, Bowlby (1969, 1973, 1980) proposed a complex theory to account for the formation of close human relationships, especially between mothers and their babies, and for what happened when these bonds were broken. He suggested that human evolution resulted in mothers and infants needing to be in close proximity for survival and that this was achieved through an interactional process involving reciprocal behaviours and feelings between mothers and babies called attachment. Temporary separation was marked by characteristic behaviours and feelings such as distress, calling, and searching. Permanent loss, such as bereavement, also triggered these feelings of intense distress and behavioural responses. Bowlby's ideas have been taken up by health and social care services, for example, in encouraging early contact between mothers and babies after birth. Bowlby's ideas were also influential in the development of Parkes's theories of loss (Parkes 1996). Both Bowlby and Parkes were psychiatrists and were in contact with patients struggling to understand the impact of their bereavements. Parkes (1971, 1993) suggested that bereavement should be considered as a major psychosocial transition, which challenged the taken-for-granted world of the bereaved person. He argued that most people think of their world as relatively stable, in which they make assumptions of perceived control. Death, especially sudden death, challenges this, as people have to adapt to changes in relationships and social status (for example from being a wife to a widow) and economic circumstances (having less money). He, like Bowlby, proposed that people progress through phases in coming to terms with their loss.

Finally, there are two well-known models that are widely applied in palliative care. Kubler-Ross (1969), a psychiatrist heavily influenced by psychoanalytic ideas, proposed a stage model of loss in relation to dying, which has been applied to bereavement. This model emphasized changing emotional expression throughout the final period of life. Worden (1982, 1991) based his therapeutic model on phases of grief and what he called 'tasks of mourning'. He suggested that grief was a process not a state and that people needed to work through their reactions to loss to achieve a complete adjustment. Of course, Parkes, Kubler-Ross, and Worden have modified and developed their ideas over time and this simple account does not do justice to the complexity of their thinking. All these theories have been critiqued and challenged, especially in relation to notions of a linear progression through phases or stages and the necessity of 'grief work' (for example, see Wortman and Silver 1989).

Stress and coping

Over the last fifty years, ideas have emerged in the psychological and medical literature about stress (Selye 1956) and coping. These ideas are based on an assumption that if certain things, called stressors, are present in sufficient amounts, they trigger a stress response. This response is both physical and psychological. Most things in our environment are within our abilities to adapt to, but it is those things that challenge this adaptation process that are considered to be stressful (Bartlett 1998). There have been a number of models proposed about how stress can be conceptualized. The most important for the purposes of this chapter is the transactional model of stress and coping developed by Lazarus and Folkman (1984). They proposed that any event may be perceived as threatening by an individual and cognitive appraisal is undertaken to estimate its degree of threat and to mobilize resources to cope with it. Coping may focus on dealing with the threat directly or may emphasize the emotional response. This is called 'problem-focused' and 'emotion-focused' coping. Stroebe and Schut (1999) developed these ideas within the context of bereavement. They proposed that, following a death, people oscillate between 'restoration-focused' coping, for example, dealing with everyday life and 'grief-focused' coping, for example, by expressing their distress. They suggest that people move between these two forms of coping with loss, although over time more coping responses become progressively more 'restoration focused'. This is called 'the dual processing model'. From these ideas they have developed therapeutic interventions to help people address both types of coping to achieve a balance.

Continuity theories

A third set of ideas have challenged notions that successful resolution of grief involves 'moving on' and 'letting go' of the deceased person. These theories are based on an assumption that people wish to maintain feelings of continuity and that, even though physical relationships may end at the time of death, these relationships become transformed but remain important within the memory of the individual and community. For example, memories of the large number of deaths that occurred during the First World War continue to haunt the UK and other countries almost 100 years after the event (Hockey 2001). Rituals to mark these losses continue to be common and some are even increasing in popularity and significance, yet few people remain alive who were present in the Trenches and witnessed these events first hand. Walter (1996, 1999) has proposed a biographical model of loss in which he suggests bereaved people seek to create a narrative that describes both the person who has died and the part they play in their lives. He argues that these narratives are socially constructed. Klass *et al.* (1996) also proposed a similar idea and illustrated this in relation to different types of loss.

Talking about loss and bereavement in primary care

Having introduced a range of theories in the previous section, we will now go on to look at how these ideas underpin the way grief and bereavement are talked about in practice. Much palliative care is delivered by general practitioners (GPs) and community nurses. It is therefore appropriate that we consider how bereavement support is provided in primary healthcare. The medicalization of bereavement and the increasing secularization of society may mean that people increasingly turn to GPs or counsellors for support following a death (Walter 1999). However, it is not clear to what extent GPs regard this as an appropriate role and even whether they have sufficient time and the appropriate expertise to engage in prolonged supportive interventions (Harris and Kendrick 1998; Main 2000). Over the last decade, there has been a rapid growth in the provision of counselling services based in or associated with UK primary healthcare. By 1999, 51 per cent of practices had counselling provision (Foster 2000). This growth has arisen from various UK government policy initiatives and recognition that the many patients who consult GPs with psychological problems may be better served by referral to those with counselling skills. However, there is evidence of great variation in the skills, training, and therapeutic approaches of counsellors employed in general practice (Wiles 1993). Dealing with loss, and more specifically bereavement, seems to form a substantial proportion of counsellors' caseloads (Sibbald *et al.* 1993). In the next section, we will draw on data from a study conducted in primary care settings in southern and south-western England (Payne *et al.* 2001)[1]. Fifty GPs and 29 counsellors took part in semi-structured interviews. We have made the assumption that how GPs and general practice-based counsellors talk about loss and bereavement reveals their understanding of these issues.

Implicit and explicit models of grief

There were a number of characteristic ways in which GPs and counsellors talked about loss and grief. There was a tension between their recognition of commonalities and generalizations versus viewing grief as a unique experience. Both GPs' and counsellors' talk indicated an implicit, and occasionally explicit, reference to models of grief based on stages and phases. They drew on models that emphasized the emotional process-ing or 'grief work' associated with loss:

> so again, I think, as (name) said, you know, you've got to go through four stages: disbelief, anger, guilt, and acceptancy' (GP 2).

We found evidence that counsellors, but not GPs, were also implicitly drawing on newer stress and coping models. The counsellor in this example uses the words 'flip over' which, in our view, demonstrates a different understanding from the 'phase and stage models' of process.

Despite the pervasiveness of the stage and phase models, there was a contradictory claim for the individuality of grief. There was a tension between the counsellors' descriptions of well-known models and their 'personal' beliefs about individual variability. This may be accounted for by two possible factors: first, their first-hand experience with bereaved people may reveal the limitations of theoretical knowledge and second, they may be drawing on postmodern social discourses which emphasize individual autonomy:

> I do think that most people's grieving process in that bit that yearning bit is so delicate and so individual (Counsellor 10).

Bereavement as a process

Bereavement was conceptualized by GPs and counsellors as a process which had two features: it was assumed to be a linear process over time and there was an assumption that people progressed from distress to resolution. They appeared to draw on a tem-plate of anticipated change, which was used to plot and compare individual progres-sion. For example, the following GP refers to 'that normal pattern' and uses this notion to 'reassure' patients. Normality in bereavement was therefore constructed as a chang-ing pattern of emotions and a decreasing display of distress:

> that normal pattern, and if I see people, and they seem to be fitting into that, and moving on a bit every so often, then I just reassure them that, yes, its ghastly, its horrible but you're moving forward, and it will get better (GP 28).

The next example demonstrates how the GP measures bereavement outcome in terms of emotional expression and draws on a template—a mental picture, to map this:

> I think it's the time factor because I have in my mind a picture of what she should be like by Christmas really, which will be gradually improving and not bursting into tears every time she comes and able to laugh and talk a bit (GP 6).

In describing this some counsellors, but not GPs, used the metaphor of a journey to describe their role in bereavement support. In the following example, counselling is explained as 'being with' the client':

> you're travelling that desperately lonely distressing road with them, you're in step, sometimes you hold their hand, if necessary (Counsellor 9).

This section has highlighted the influence of language and discourses of grief and loss used by GPs and counsellors. We have argued that the stage and phase models remain the most important way in which grief is talked about, although GPs and counsellors acknowledged their caution in not making assumptions about the universality of stages or their linear progression. The template provided by models of grief (usually a stage model) was a powerful device, used by GPs and counsellors to map and identify patterns of 'normal' and 'abnormal' grieving. More recent understanding of loss based on stress and coping theory and biographical integration have yet to become common discourses although helping clients to tell the story was a common counselling strategy. While the majority of terms and, we would argue, conceptual understandings are shared by GPs and counsellors, we noted a few differences mostly in how they viewed their role. Some GPs talked of certain types of people being 'at risk' or vulnerable, for example, following suicide or the death of a child. General practitioners used these notions of 'riskiness' to guide their interpretation of possible abnormal reactions. Some counsellors talked of bereaved people 'getting stuck', that is, not moving through the process of grief. They described how they identified 'being stuck' and the strategies they used to 'move' people onward. We suggest that some GPs felt relatively powerless to support bereaved people because they construed bereavement support as requiring both large amounts of time to talk and counselling skills. Counselling—a 'talking therapy'—seemed an appropriate response, as it requires people to do their 'grief work' predominantly through talk. Thus we would argue that GPs saw their role as screening for 'abnormal' or 'risky' bereavements and that counsellors' interactions with clients focused on encouraging and enabling clients to 'talk' their way to an agreed and, we would suggest, socially constructed understanding of loss.

Bereavement support in specialist palliative care

Hospice philosophy encompasses the care of patients and their families, which continues after death into the bereavement period. The majority of UK hospices regard the provision of bereavement support as integral to their services, although there is less consensus about the nature of the services that should be provided and how they should be delivered or allocated (Wilkes 1993; Payne and Relf 1994). It has been argued that, for a number of reasons, bereavement support has been the least well-developed aspect of hospices and specialist palliative care services (Payne and Relf 1994; Payne 2001a). Most services are based on an assumption that bereavement is a major stressful life event and that a minority of people experience substantial disruption to their physical, psychological, and social functioning (Parkes 1996). Parkes (1993) has argued that offering support to people who have adequate internal and external resources can be disempowering and detrimental to coping. There are few methodologically rigorous evaluations of general bereavement support services and even less in relation to hospices (Payne et al. 1999).

There is much that we do not know about what happens in hospice bereavement services and what constitutes good practice. Services have tended to be set up and run outside formal disciplinary boundaries. This means that it is predominantly nurses, social workers, counsellors, chaplains, and perhaps psychologists who have been involved, with less input from medical staff than in other aspects of specialist palliative care services. In many services volunteers play an important role in supporting bereaved people. Volunteers may enhance the range of services offered and address the need to make services culturally appropriate by involving local people and those from different minority ethnic groups. However, there is controversy about the extent to which volunteer labour is valued and how the needs of volunteer workers are met (Payne 2001b). Volunteers require recruitment, selection, training, and supervision. Relf (1998) has pointed out that providing for the needs of volunteer workers in bereavement support is a demanding and skilled activity.

Bereavement support may include a broad range of activities such as social evenings, befriending, one-to-one counselling, and support groups. Bereavement support may start before the death, when families are put in touch with volunteer workers who may befriend them and maintain contact with them into the bereavement period. Such services offer the opportunity for relationships to be built up over time and for newly bereaved people to be spared the difficulty of making new relationships when they are at their most vulnerable. However, most bereavement services only offer postdeath contact and support. It might be most helpful to consider bereavement support in three broad categories, as shown in Table 10.1. Readers may be aware of other activities that are offered in their own services. Of course, there may be considerable overlap in the aims and delivery of some of these activities. For example, a drop-in centre might enable a bereaved person to talk one to one with a social worker, which may be perceived as therapeutic. Likewise, a bereaved person may agree to attend an art therapy programme because it enables them to get out of the house and meet new people, which is a predominantly social outcome.

All bereavement services need to set up systems to allocated clients and most have to make decisions about their use of resources. There are formal ways, such as using questionnaires and checklists, to assess how likely it is that a bereaved person will have an adverse outcome. There are well-recognized attributes of the person, their environment, and the nature of the death that allow predictions to be made about which people need help (Saunders 1993). This is called risk assessment. For example, a person with previous mental health problems experiencing concurrent losses, such as their job or home and witnessing a traumatic sudden death of their young child in a car accident, is likely to be more vulnerable than a person bereaved of their elderly

Table 10.1 Types of hospice and specialist palliative care bereavement support for adults

Social activities	Supportive activities	Therapeutic activities
Condolence cards	Drop-in centre/ coffee mornings	One-to-one counselling with
Anniversary (of death) cards	Self-help groups	professional or trained volunteer
Bereavement information leaflets	Information support groups	Therapeutic support groups
Bereavement information resources (videos/books)	Volunteer visiting or befriending	Drama, music, or art therapy
		Relaxation classes
Staff attending the funeral		Complementary therapies
Social evenings		Psychotherapy
Memorial services or other rituals		

grandmother after a chronic illness. Although risk-assessment measures are available, none are perfect and most services allocate bereavement support based on clinical judgement (Payne and Relf 1994). Hospice bereavement support services also need to be able to identify when clients present such difficult and complex problems that they exceed their capacity to deal with them. Close and well-established links with other services, such as liaison psychiatric, clinical psychology, and specialist bereavement support services (for example, suicide support groups) are needed.

The emotional demands placed on those who witness grief and support the bereaved require skill, knowledge, and sensitivity. The paradoxical nature of bereavement support, which requires both professional standards of knowledge and skill and the warmth of human understanding and sensitivity, represents a challenge for all. There is a dilemma in training volunteers and professionals that the compassion and empathy that lead them into this work becomes constrained by a framework imposed by models of bereavement. We have seen in the previous section how general practice-based counsellors helped to shape their clients bereavement experience. Of course, we lacked data from their clients to demonstrate the extent to which counsellors' versions of reality were in fact imposed or resisted by their clients. However, exposure to repeated distress needs to be acknowledged as potentially difficult to deal with. It is generally considered to be good practice to ensure that supervision is available to bereavement care workers, in which emotional off-loading and discussion of difficult situations can be dealt with on a regular basis (Payne *et al.* 1999).

Children and bereavement

Tom, aged 8 and Jake, aged 6, knew there was something wrong with their dad. They had noticed over the past year that he no longer took them out and that he stayed in bed for quite a lot of the time. One Saturday morning they were told that as a special treat (although it was not school holidays) they were going to stay for a week or two with their aunt and uncle some 50 miles away. When mum came to collect them nearly two weeks later, they were told that dad had died and that he had gone to a special place. The funeral had taken place the day before they returned home. Initially both children were surprised (and delighted!) by all the attention they were getting. They were always being invited to stay with friends or to go home with school friends for tea and had never had so many visits to the cinema or MacDonalds. Six months later the invitations and treats had all but stopped. Jake was bedwetting and Tom's behaviour at school had changed from a little boy who worked hard to one who was rude, disruptive, and at times violent to other children.

The above case history illustrates some of the difficulties that families face when a parent is diagnosed with a terminal illness. Should the children be told what is happening and if so how and when should they be told and who should tell them? Should they be present at the death and be involved in the funeral?

Support prior to the death

Each year, two per cent of all children are bereaved of a parent before the age of 18 years—many of these deaths are sudden, for example, due to accident or sudden cardiac death but a significant number may be due to terminal illness. How can children be helped around the dying process and their bereavement? It is known that children whose parents die from cancer, where there is often time to prepare the child and family, have fewer psychological difficulties than children whose parents die suddenly, for example, suicide (Pfeffer *et al.* 2000). It can be difficult to involve a child during the parent's illness. The surviving parent in a desperate bid to spare the children the pain they themselves are facing, may act similarly to the mother in the case history above and may be coerced into doing so by other family members in the belief that they are protecting and helping the child. However these actual mechanisms may not be protective and whilst delaying the initial pain do not spare children from later distress or the reality of what has happened.

Additionally, the sick parent may be so unwell as to be unable to tolerate the child for any length of time and sometimes parents may withdraw from the family during the latter stages of the illness, again making it difficult for children to have any meaningful interaction. Encouraging children to visit for short periods and to write stories or draw pictures may be one method of keeping them involved. Older children will have more real understanding of what is happening. All children however need to be reassured that whatever happened they would be loved and cared for. This can be difficult, as often the partner is so involved in caring for the dying parent that they may not have the emotional capacity or the time to give to the children. Increasing numbers of children grow up in single-parent families and for them, the prospect of losing their only parent is enormous. The mobilization of extended family resources is necessary to all for the future and to support the child who may be the caregiver to the dying parent (Segal and Simkins 1993).

Children who experience sudden, unexpected bereavement are thought to be at a higher risk of developing problems. For those who have witnessed traumatic events such as accidents or suicide, there may be residual horrific images to contend with and for a minority, posttraumatic stress disorder may occur (Cerel *et al.* 1999). Christ (2000) studied the experiences of 88 families and their 157 children throughout the six months of a parent's terminal illness due to cancer and for 14 months after the death. Her analysis indicates that children reacted in ways that were heavily influenced by their developmental stage at the time of their loss. She also proposed that childhood loss should not be conceptualized as a single event, because it tended to precipitate a cascade of events bought about by the experience of illness on family functioning, the transition from dual to single parenting, and the possible subsequent remarriage of their remaining parent and the formation of a new family. Each of these events are challenging in their own right but bereaved children are often faced with a multitude of changes that may challenge their coping resources. Therefore, psychological and other responses to bereavement may be triggered by any one or a combination of these challenges as children grow to adulthood.

Support after death

It is widely believed that where possible it is helpful if children are able to attend the funeral if they so wish and also, if they wish, to be involved in the actual service itself. It is important however for a child to have an accompanying adult and to be reassured that they can leave at any time they wish—the surviving parent may be so overcame by their own grief as to be unable to support the children during the funeral. Encouraging children to draw pictures or to write a story or letter that can be placed in the coffin can also help the child in the process of saying goodbye. There is still a belief that children do not understand the meaning of death but research has suggested that children as young as five or six years old have a clear concept of what death means (Lansdown and Benjamin 1985). Following a longitudinal study of bereaved children in the USA and Israel, Silverman (2000) has argued that even very young children can be helped by being given a clear explanation about what is happening when a family member dies. Children need to be told about what has happened in a language that they can understand (Black 1998). Euphemisms such as 'passed away' or 'gone to sleep' should be avoided. Children often have many questions regarding the terminal illness, for example, 'What is cancer?' or 'What is chemotherapy?'; again these questions need to be answered in a language that children can understand and the support of a doctor who is willing to discuss such questions with children is invaluable (Monroe and Kraus 1996; Thompson and Payne 2000).

Do all bereaved children need support? Harrington and Harrison (1999) describes a plethora of counselling services and at present no evidence to suggest which, if any, are of value for the bereaved child and their family. Evaluating the effectiveness of such services is difficult especially as outcomes, for example, reduction of psychiatric morbidity can only be assessed several years later (Stokes *et al.* 1997). Most professionals would agree that all bereaved children should be given the opportunity to talk about the death and to explore and share their feelings (Blanche and Smith 2000; Carroll and Griffin 1977). Children however do not grieve constantly and may dip in and out of intense grief for very short time periods. This can be difficult for family members to deal with alongside their own grief. Our case history illustrated how problems can be minimized during the first few months following a death when family and friends rally round and provide support. Lloyd-Williams *et al.* (1998) found that the peak time for children to present to the GP following the death of a parent was 4.8 months and these presentations were frequently for somatic symptoms for which no organic causes could be found. This probably reflects the time when the attention of others is decreasing and when the reality of the loss may overwhelm the surviving parent causing strained relationships within the family.

Several models of bereavement support groups for children have been suggested (Mulcahey and Young 1995; Christ *et al.* 1991; Zambelli *et al.* 1988). A recent survey of 107 childhood bereavement services in the UK identified that 85 per cent of childhood bereavement services were located within the voluntary sector; 14 per cent were dedicated childhood bereavement services whilst 86 per cent were located within another organization, 44 per cent of these being hospices (Rolls and Payne in press). The majority of services (71 per cent) took referral for any child, the remaining 27 per cent only offered services if the family members had died in their care. Most services (72.5 per cent) relied on both paid and unpaid staff with 115 relying entirely on paid staff and 14.3 per cent relying entirely on unpaid staff. The interventions offered ranged from individual family work (85.7 per cent) to individual child work (61.5 per cent), group work with families (52.7 per cent), and group work with children (45.1 per cent). In addition services offered prebereavement support (63.7 per cent), a 'drop-in' service (16.5 per cent), information and advice (94.5 per cent), training (31.9 per cent), and the provision resources (87.9 per cent). In addition to offering a service to children and their families, 75 per cent of childhood bereavement services provided a service to secondary users, for example, schools (70 per cent), emergency services (27.5 per cent), and other professionals (63 per cent).

Winston's wish is an example of a child bereavement programme in the UK that focuses on providing support and informing those closest to the child, for example, teachers, nursing, and care staff as to how to help a child through their grief (Stokes *et al.* 1999). Children who are bereaved may feel very isolated—they may be the only children who have been bereaved within their school, for example, causing them to feel stigmatized and very alone. The weekend camps are aimed at bringing bereaved children together to meet others in a similar situation and to give them an opportunity to tell their story, to ask questions, to have fun, and to encourage them to think of life in the future, which for many children bereaved of a parent, may include a stepparent. One of the key aims of the programme is to help parents to support their children, for example, by encouraging children to talk about the deceased parent and sharing memories—'Do you remember when ...' (Nickman *et al.* 1998).

A bereaved child may experience the grieving process at several different time points, many years after the death, at major milestones in their lives (Baker *et al.* 1992; Lohnes and Kalter 1994). This chapter has aimed to discuss some of the issues that are important for those working within palliative care in seeking to provide support for bereaved children. The last words should go to those we are trying to help:

> ... In the days after she had gone, I had mixed emotions ... at times I felt pathetic like if only I hadn't hidden all those sandwiches, if only I hadn't answered back all those times ... At other times I would think she hadn't gone, it's only we can't touch her or see her and we'll always, always love her and as my Gran told me, the sadness will go eventually and I believe her ...

Notes

1. Data for this chapter are drawn from a National Health Service Executive South West Research and Development-funded research project, concerned with exploring counselling for the bereaved in primary care. We wish to acknowledge the contribution of the GPs and other members of the research team—Dr Rose Wiles, Professor David Field, and Dr Nikki Jarrett—to this study. We also wish to acknowledge Izzie for allowing us to share her feelings at her mum's death.

References

Baker J, Sedney M, Gross E (1992). Psychological tasks for bereaved children. *Am J Orthopsychiat* **62:**105–16.

Bartlett D (1998). *Stress.* Buckingham: Open University Press.

Black D (1998). Bereavement in childhood. *BMJ* **316:**931–3.

Blanche M, Smith S (2000). Bereaved children's support groups: where are we now? *Eur J Palliative Care* **7:**142–4.

Bowlby J (1969). *Attachment and loss. Vol. 1. Attachment.* London: Hogarth Press.

Bowlby J (1973). *Attachment and loss. Vol. 2. Separation.* London: Hogarth Press.

Bowlby J (1980). *Attachment and loss. Vol. 3. Loss: sadness and depression.* London: Hogarth Press.

Carroll M, Griffin R (1997). Reaffirming life's puzzle: support for bereaved children. *Am J Hospice Palliative Care* **14:**231–5.

Cerel J, Fristed M, Weller E, Weller R (1999). Suicide-bereaved children and adolescents: a controlled longitudinal examination. *J Am Acad Paediat Adolescent Psychiat* **38:**672–9.

Christ G (2000). *Healing children's grief: surviving a parent's death from cancer.* New York: Oxford University Press.

Christ G, Siegel K, Mesagno F, Langosch D (1991). A preventative intervention program for bereaved children: problems of implementation. *Am J Orthopsychiat* **61:**168–78.

Fenichel O (1945). *The psychoanalytic theory of neurosis.* New York: Norton.

Firth S (2001). Hindu death and mourning rituals: the impact of geographic mobility. In: Hockey J, Katz J, Small N (ed.). *Grief, mourning and death ritual.* Buckingham: Open University Press. pp. 237–46.

Foster J (2000). Counselling in primary care and the new NHS. *Br J Guidance Counselling* **28:**175–90.

Freud S (1917). *Mourning and melancholia.* London: Hogarth Press.

Harrington R, Harrison L (1999). Unproven assumptions about the imapct of bereavement on children. *J Royal Soc Med* **92:**230–3.

Harris T, Kendrick T (1998). Bereavement care in general practice: a survey in South Thames region. *Br J Gen Pract* **48:**1560–4.

Hockey J (2001). Changing death rituals. In: Hockey J, Katz J, Small N (ed.). *Grief, mourning and death ritual.* Buckingham: Open University Press. pp. 185–211.

Hockey J, Katz J, Small N (2001). *Grief, mourning and death ritual.* Buckingham: Open University Press.

Klass D, Silverman PR, Nickman SL (1996). *Continuing bonds.* Philadephia: Taylor and Francis.

Kubler-Ross E (1969). *On death and dying.* New York: Macmillan.

Lansdown R, Benjamin C (1985). The development of the concept of death in children aged 5–9. *Child Care Health Develop* **11**:13–20.

Lazarus RS, Folkman S (1984). *Stress, appraisal and coping.* New York: Springer.

Lindemann E (1944). Symptomatology and management of acute grief. *Am J Psychiat* **101**:141–8.

Lloyd-Williams M, Wilkinson C, Lloyd-Williams F (1998). Do bereaved children consult the primary care team more frequently? *Eur J Cancer Care* **7**:120–4.

Lohnes K, Kalter N (1994). Preventative intervention groups for parentally bereaved children. *Am J Orthopsychiat* **64**:594–603.

Main J (2000). Improving management of bereavement in general practice based on a survey of recently bereaved subjects in a single general practice. *Br J Gen Pract* **50**:863–6.

Monroe B, Kraus F (1996). Children and loss. *Br J Hosp Med* **56**:260–4.

Mulcahey AM (1995). A bereavement support group for children. *Cancer Pract* **3**:150–6.

Nickman S, Silverman P, Normand C (1998). Children's construction of a deceased parent: the surviving parent's contribution. *Am J Orthopsychiat* **68**:126–34.

Oxford English dictionary. 2nd edn (1989). Oxford: Oxford University Press.

Parkes CM (1971). Psychosocial transitions: a field for study. *Soc Sci Med* **5**:101–14.

Parkes CM (1993). Bereavement as a psychosocial transition: processes of adaptation to change. In: Stroebe MS, Stroebe W, Hansson RO (ed.). *Handbook of bereavement.* Cambridge: Cambridge University Press. pp. 91–101.

Parkes CM (1996). *Bereavement.* 3rd edn. London: Routledge.

Parkes CM, Laungani P, Young B (ed.) (1997). *Death and bereavement across cutlures.* London: Routledge.

Payne S (2001*a*). Bereavement support: something for everyone? *Int J Palliative Nursing* **7**:108.

Payne S (2001*b*). The role of volunteers in hospice bereavement support in New Zealand. *Palliative Med* **15**:107–15.

Payne S, Relf M (1994). The assessment of need for bereavement follow-up in palliative and hospice care. *Palliative Med* **8**:291–7.

Payne S, Horn S, Relf M (1999). *Loss and bereavement.* Buckingham: Open University Press.

Payne S, Wiles R, Field D, Jarrett N (2001). Counselling the bereaved in general practice. London: National Health Service Executive South East; final report.

Pfeffer C, Karus D, Siegel K (2000). Child survivors of parental death from cancer or suicide: depressive behavioural outcomes. *Psycho-oncology* **9**:1–10.

Relf M (1998). Involving volunteers in bereavement counselling. *EurJ Palliative Care* **5**:61–5.

Rolls E, Payne S (in press). Childhood bereavement services: a survey of UK provision. *Palliative Med.*

Saunders CM (1993). Risk factors in bereavement outcome. In: Stroebe MS, Stroebe W, Hansson RO (ed.). *Handbook of bereavement.* Cambridge: Cambridge University Press. pp. 255–70.

Segal J, Simkins J (1993). *My mum needs me: helping children with ill or disabled parents .* London: Penguin.

Selye H (1956). *The stress of life.* New York: McGraw-Hill.

Sibbald B, Addington-Hall L, Brenneman D, Freeling P (1993). Counsellors in English and Welsh general practices: their nature and distribution. *BMJ* **306**:29–33.

Silverman P (2000). *Never too young to know.* New York: Oxford University Press.

Small N (2001). Theories of grief: a critical review. In: Hockey J, Katz J, Small N (ed.). *Grief, mourning and death ritual*. Buckingham: Open University Press. pp. 19–48.

Stokes J, Wyer S, Crossley D (1997). The challenge of evaluating a child bereavement programme. *Palliative Med* **11**:179–90.

Stokes J, Pennington J, Monroe B, Papadatou D, Relf M (1999). Developing services for bereaved children: a discussion of the theoretical and practical issues involved. *Mortality* **4**:291–307.

Stroebe M, Schut H (1999). The dual process model of coping with bereavement: rationale and description. *Death Stud* **23**:197–224.

Sullivan HL (1956). The dynamics of emotion. In: Sullivan HL (ed.). *Clinical studies in psychiatry*. New York: Norton.

Thompson F, Payne S (2000). Bereaved children's questions to a doctor. *Mortality* **5**:74–96.

Walter T (1996). A new model of grief: bereavement and biography. *Mortality* **1**:1–29.

Walter T (1999). *On bereavement*. Buckingham: Open University Press.

Wiles R (1993). *Counselling in general practice*. Southampton: Institute for Health Policy Studies, University of Southampton.

Wilkes E (1993). Characteristics of hospice bereavement services. *J Cancer Care* **2**:183–9.

Worden JW (1982). *Grief counselling and grief therapy: a handbook for the mental health practitioner*. New York: Springer.

Worden JW (1991). *Grief counselling and grief therapy*. 2nd edn. New York: Springer.

Wortman CB, Silver RC (1989). The myths of coping with loss. *J Consulting Clin Psychol* **57**:349–57.

Zambelli G, Lcark E, Barile L, de Jong A (1988). An interdisciplinary approach to clinical intervention for childhood bereavement. *Death Stud* **12**:41–50.

Chapter 11

Staff stress, suffering, and compassion in palliative care

Mary LS Vachon and Ruth Benor

Introduction

Caring for patients and their families facing terminal illness can be both stressful and rewarding for the healthcare practitioner. Caregivers frequently feel that in their compassion they are truly suffering with the client and that they may become overwhelmed.

This chapter will review the personal and environmental factors that may interact and cause stress in palliative care and also discuss the issues of suffering and compassion and suggest coping strategies to avoid becoming overwhelmed. The chapter will explore ways in which caregivers may be able to derive a deep personal satisfaction in their work without succumbing to burn-out and compassion fatigue.

No matter what stressor is experienced, whether it is unique to the individual or arises within the clinical environment, the need to survive and to survive well is a basic instinct. In understanding responses to stressors it is important to realize that living systems do not function mechanically and do not operate in isolated parts (Haigh 2002). The process of life is complex and arises out of the inextricable intertwining of subtle relationships between structures, patterns, and their processes (Bartol and Courts 2000). It is important to raise awareness of the nature of stress and its potential to compromise the individual as one seeks to practice within such an emotionally challenging field as palliative care (Benor 1996).

The healthcare practitioner cannot be separated from their personality, their unique history or responses to stress, and their own perceptions.

Personal variables

Demographic variables

Age

Younger caregivers have been found to report more stressors, more manifestations of stress, and fewer coping strategies (Vachon 1987). Younger physicians reported higher degrees of burn-out (Deckard *et al.* 1994) and in a UK study of oncologists and palliative care physicians, burn-out was associated with being under the age of 55 (Ramirez *et al.* 1995). Increased job satisfaction was found to be associated with older age (Beck-Friis *et al.* 1993), although older staff members may be more sensitive to a gap between their real and ideal work situation and, if such a gap occurs, older care-givers might be more vulnerable to stress reactions (Bram and Katz 1989).

Gender

Gender has also been found to influence response to stressors in the workplace. At Memorial Sloan–Kettering Cancer Center (MSKCC) (Kash *et al.* 2000) women oncology house staff and nurses had the highest level of emotional exhaustion and psychological distress on the Maslach Burnout Scale (Maslach and Jackson 1986) when staff physicians, house staff, and nurses were compared.

Women physicians were found to experience more role strain than their men counterparts (Heim 1991) and were more likely to report suicidal ideation (Cassels 1993). In a large study of almost 2000 UK family practitioners (Cooper *et al.* 1989), men physicians had higher anxiety scores than the norms, had less job satisfaction, and drank more alcohol than their women counterparts. Dealing with death and dying was not a major source of stress; however it was associated with excess alcohol use, especially for women physicians. While experiencing more role strain, women physicians have also been found to report greater job satisfaction and greater well-being than matched controls (Cooper *et al.* 1989). The latter finding was replicated in the more recent Physician Worklife Study (McMurray *et al.* 2000). Women were more likely than their men colleagues to report satisfaction with their specialty and with patient and colleague relationships but less likely to be satisfied with autonomy, relationships with community, pay, and resources. Women physicians were also more likely to report less work control than their men counterparts regarding day-to-day aspects of practice, including volume of patient load. In addition they were less well paid. A lack of support and higher degrees of burn-out in women physicians may well play as crucial a role as work and family issues in leading women physicians to experience difficulty with 'fit' in particular settings and leading possibly to the fact that women physicians are likely to work fewer hours, retire earlier, and be inactive during part of their medical career (McMurray *et al.* 2000).

Personality

Hospice workers have been found to ground their work in self-awareness and a clear personal philosophy (Zerwekh 1993). Working with dying patients has been found to shape one's attitude toward death and dying (Alexander and Ritchie 1990). Those who coped adequately with death were found to have a tendency to live in the present, rather than the past or the future. They scored higher on inner-directedness, self-actualizing value, existentiality, spontaneity, self-regard, self-acceptance, acceptance of aggression, and capacity for intimate contact (Robbins 1991).

Hardiness. The personality characteristic of hardiness, which consists of commitment, control, and challenge (Kobasa 1979; Kobasa *et al.* 1982) was associated with decreased burn-out in American nurses (Simoni and Paterson 1997) and Greek oncology nurses (Papadatou *et al.* 1994) and with less demoralization in the MSKCC study (Kash *et al.* 2000). The sense of control over things that happen in life and in the work environment was found to protect nurses from emotional exhaustion, depersonalization, and a lack of personal accomplishment. Nurses who experienced higher degrees of burn-out reported a lack of a sense of control over external events (Papadatou *et al.* 1994).

In a study of 1925 white- and blue-collar university employees in Australia (Sharpley *et al.* 1995), 'cognitive hardiness', which assesses involvement, challenge, and control (Nowack 1990) was found to be the best predictor of the ability to manage job stress, anxiety, daily hassles, and to maintain a healthy lifestyle. Hardy behaviours depend on both behavioural competence and supportive environments. These variables allow the individual to find the resources essential to coping, to make use of social networks when needed, and to transform stressful experiences into meaningful experiences (Bowsher and Keep 1995). Stressors are seen as manageable by those who are hardy (Simoni and Paterson 1997).

Sense of control. The issue of control is not a simple one. Shapiro *et al.* (1996) wrote of the positive and negative aspects of controlling ourselves and our world. They use the illustration from the *Bible*, of Cain and Abel. When Cain was told by God to master his emotions he did not 'practice deep breathing and use cognitive coping strategies to regain a sense of control; (nor) did he reframe and reappraise the situation in order to keep a perspective–retrospective control, decisional control, and interpretive secondary control'. Instead he exerted decisional and behavioural control by killing his brother!

Such control efforts should also be directed toward generativity, compassionate service for the healing of others, and interpersonal and collective well-being.

Spirituality and religious belief systems

Spiritual and religious belief systems have been found to be helpful in oncology and palliative care (Vachon 1995). A sense of spirituality can be helpful to caregivers as they struggle to find meaning in the work they are doing (Vachon 2001; Heim 1991). It has been said that burn-out has very little to do with work or overwork but occurs because of the caregiver having lost the ability to manage pain well and to keep balance in their life. Being truly spiritual involved having a real balance in one's life (D'Shano 1996).

Nurses attracted to hospice work have been found to be more religious than others (Vachon 1995; Amenta 1984). Compared with oncology nurses, hospice nurses reported a greater sense of personal spirituality, more frequent spiritual caregiving, and more positive perspectives regarding spiritual caregiving (Taylor *et al.* 1999).

In the MSKCC study nurses were more religious than other groups. Those who described being extremely religious had significantly lower scores on diminished empathy or depersonalization and lower emotional exhaustion on the Maslach Burnout scale (Maslach and Jackson 1982; Maslach and Jackson 1986; Kash *et al.* 2000).

For many caregivers a spiritual or religious philosophy, centred on a commitment to serve others, may be both helpful and key to deriving a sense of meaning in difficult times (Vachon 1987). Remen (1996) speaks of the power of a personal sense of meaning to change the experience of work, of relationships, and even of life:

> Meaning may become a very practical matter for those of us who do difficult work or lead difficult lives and is a strength. Physicians often seek their strength in competence. Indeed, competence and expertise are two of the most respected qualities in the medical subculture, as well as in our society. But important as they are, they are not sufficient to fully sustain us … Competence may bring us satisfaction. Finding meaning in a familiar task often allows us to go beyond this and find in the most routine of tasks a deep sense of joy and even gratitude.

Stressors in palliative care

Stressors in the palliative care environment derive from three major categories of stressors: the work environment, variables related to one's occupational role, and issues related to the patients and families with whom one works (Vachon 1987). Work in palliative care can be described as emotional labour, which is 'the labor involved in dealing with other people's feelings, a core component of which is the regulation of emotions' (James 1989). This work is often performed by women. Such work also involves the regulation of emotion between the carer and the person being cared for, which is one of the sometimes tremendous but rewarding challenges of work in palliative care.

When Swedish nurses working in hospice and oncology were compared (Rasmussen and Sandman 2000) the content and quality of the nurses' physical and emotional labour differed significantly. Hospice nurses spent significantly more of their time with patients and relatives (37 per cent) than oncology nurses did (21 per cent). When they were with patients, most of the nurses' care involved physical activities such as helping patients with their daily activities in the hospice and helping patients with needs in relation to investigations and treatment in the oncology unit. The emotional labour of talking with patients and providing emotional support consumed 9 per cent of the hospice nurses' time and 4 per cent of the oncology nurses' time. The proportion of direct care time taken up by emotional labour was 19 per cent for the oncology nurses and 24 per cent for the hospice nurses. The authors compare this study with observational studies in an oncology unit in Denmark (Hansen 1995) and an acute and long-term care unit in Sweden (Franssén 1997). In both of the studies, the investigators found a discrepancy between the nurses' thoughts and actions. In their communications the nurses were dedicated to patient-oriented and holistic care but in their actions they prioritized routinized tasks or social and professional interactions with colleagues. During quiet working days, rather than engaging in the emotional labour to which they were committed, the nurses utilized their time other ways. It was hypothesized that this was a way of the nurses maintaining control.

Role overload

In a study involving a random sample of hospice nurses throughout the USA, job pressure involving on call duty, the need to travel to patients, and repeated crises was one of the least appealing aspects of hospice nursing (Amenta 1995). Hospice initially prided itself on having the time to take to spend with patients and their families. As financial constraints have grown, hospice nurses are finding themselves more and more stretched to provide the type of care they want to provide (Vachon 2001).

Role conflict

Role conflict in palliative care can evolve from a variety of sources when one's role as a team member is in conflict with what one thinks might be in the best interest of patients. Such issues include conflict about end-of-life care between nurses and physicians; conflict with patients who may not yet be ready to accept the reality of impending death, when the nurse feels it is time for them to stop aggressive treatment (Kuuppelomäki and Lauri 1998); 'allowing' patients to maintain control, while feeling disappointed in not being able to fully discuss patients' expressed wishes to die; taking actions to help patients or families maintain a sense of control, while questioning the wisdom and morality of their decisions; dealing with the sometimes hazy distinction between patient autonomy and a professional ethic of care (Hart *et al.* 1998); and the decision to transfer patients from active treatment settings to hospice or palliative care programmes primarily for economic reasons (Byock 1998). Inexperienced nurses caring for very symptomatic palliative care patients in the community may feel role conflict between the patient's right to good symptom control and the nurse's fear of hastening the patient's death (Coyle 1997).

Hart *et al.* (1998) used critical incidents from the practice of palliative care nurses to improve skills in psychosocial care. They found that in the practice incidents that nurses identified, they repeatedly related roles in which they were mediating in a conflict situation in order to restore harmony and control. The nurses reported difficulty with patients who chose not to communicate their feelings about death and dying with either staff or their families and those who chose not to take medications in order that death might come more quickly. Patients' actions to take 'personal control' of their situation and to refuse palliative care threatened the nurses' feelings about their role and function as palliative care nurses and made them feel they had not been good enough advocates for palliative care.

Team conflict

Team communication problems have been a significant part of hospice, palliative care, and to a lesser extent oncology since the early days of these specialties (Vachon 2000). A lack of support from one's team members is associated with high levels of depression (Bené and Foxall 1991). Organizational factors, such as personality issues and team conflict, were more commonly reported stressors than were problems in dealing with patients and families and issues related to death and dying (Vachon 1987).

A more recent study of hospice nurses in the UK (Payne 2001) found that dealing with death and dying, inadequate preparation, and workload were slightly more problematic than were conflict with doctors, conflict with other nurses, lack of support, and uncertainty concerning treatment. However, in that study conflict with staff contributed to both the emotional exhaustion and depersonalization sub-scales of the Maslach Burnout Inventory (Maslach and Jackson 1986).

Issues of death and dying

The most problematic stressor reported by hospice nurses and nursing assistants with an average of 5.7 years in hospice care (Payne 2001) was death and dying. Patients coming to terms with dying was the main death-related concern of nurses working in acute care, hospice, and community settings (Copp and Dunn, 1993) and in palliative care (Alexander and Ritchie, 1990). There can also be difficulties when patients do not want to die in the way nurses feel they 'should' die (Hart *et al.* 1998).

The difficulties associated with the care of dying persons may in part be due to the close connections palliative care nurses often develop with their patients. Whereas traditionally nurses and other professionals have been taught to maintain a boundary between themselves and their clients, in palliative care and oncology very close relationships can and do develop (Trygstad 1986).

Multiple loss

One does not have to work very long in palliative care before one begins to feel the accumulation of grief related to the experience of multiple loss. Although Mount had written of the concept of multiple loss within the context of oncology (Mount 1986), the concept became more recognized with the AIDS epidemic. The concept of multiple loss in AIDS caregivers reflected in part the reality that many caregivers were caring for dying patients, while partners, friends, and members of their social network were dying at the same time (Vachon 2001).

Caregivers in palliative care may be caring for many patients who die within a short time of one another. This grief can accumulate over the years leading to significant depression. Multiple losses may also result in chronic grief because there is no time to finish grieving for one loss before another one occurs and 'multiple loss syndrome' includes the effects of chronic, anticipatory, and unresolved grief, as well as the compounding effects of experiencing several episodes of grief concurrently (Cho and Cassidy 1994).

These losses may extend beyond the deaths of patients. Papadatou (2000) has defined the losses as

(1) loss of a close relationship with a particular patient;

(2) loss due to the professional's identification with the pain of family members;

(3) loss of one's unmet goals and expectations;

(4) losses related to one's personal system of beliefs and assumptions about life;

(5) past unresolved losses or anticipated future losses;

(6) the death of self.

Finding coping styles to deal with the grief inherent in palliative care that fit with one's professional style can minimize burn-out. Remen (1996) speaks of the dangers of professionals getting locked into their sometimes rigid ways of coping: 'One of the reasons many physicians feel drained by their work is that they do not know how to make an opening to receive anything from their patients'. She notes that the tendency of healthcare professionals to protect themselves from loss and grief, rather than grieving and healing their losses is one of the major causes of burn-out.

Suffering and compassion

As is clear from the above, there are numerous sources of stress in palliative care, yet the work can be very rewarding and evidence generally indicates that the stress is less than that experienced in other settings (Vachon 1995). However, constant exposure to the suffering of others can take its toll. Traditionally religions have attempted to deal with the issue of suffering: 'It is sometimes said that suffering is at once the central puzzle of and a basic reason for religion' (Little 1989). Western religions tend to frame suffering as a 'problem'. How could a good and loving God permit His people to suffer? Eastern religions tend to see suffering as a 'mystery' (Gregory and Russell 1999). Buddhism teaches the Four Noble Truths (Longaker 1997):

(1) knowing that suffering pervades our existence;

(2) discovering the cause of our suffering;

(3) understanding that we can bring an end to suffering;

(4) entering the path which enables us to become free of suffering.

Suffering work is felt by both those who suffer and those who would help. Both the sufferer and the helper must grasp what is involved, what works, for there is a difference between suffering that leads to health and suffering that destroys (Emerson 1986).

In the face of suffering, caregivers are often filled with a sense of compassion. The dictionary says that to feel compassion is to experience a feeling of deep sympathy and sorrow for another who is stricken by suffering or misfortune, accompanied by a strong desire to alleviate the pain or to remove its cause (Stein 1967). To feel compassion is to suffer with another person—the key to sustaining ourselves in the arena of palliative care is to learn how to feel compassion while maintaining the delicate boundary that keeps us from being destroyed by our work.

Watson (1989), a nurse theoretician, states that

> When both care providers and care receiver are co-participants in caring, the release can allow the one who is cared for to be the one who cares, through the reflection of the human condition that in turn nourishes the humanness of the care provider. In such connectedness they are both capable of transcending self, time and space.

Fox (1999) writes of the image of the man in sapphire blue that was received by the twelfth-century mystic, Hildegard of Bingen. Fox notes that the colour of the heart chakra is green. Hildegard built her entire theology on viriditas or 'greening power'. She felt that all creatures contained the greening power of the Holy Spirit, which made all things creative and nourishing. In her picture of the man in sapphire blue, the man's hands are outstretched in front of his chest. This gesture is an ancient metaphor for compassion because compassion is about taking heart energy and putting it into one's hands—that is putting it to work in the world. This is the work of healing and assisting.

> An energy field surrounds the man. Clearly this is a man whose "body is in the soul" and not whose soul is in the body. In the illumination there is an aperture at the man's head, so that this powerful healing energy can leave his own field and mix with others-and vice versa. (Fox 1999)

Psychoneuroimmunology and stress

Psychoneuroimmunology (PNI) strives to demonstrate the complexities of connections, in particular aimimg to identify the casual pathways through which the stress–health link is mediated (Bartlett 1998) and it investigates the interactions between the neuroendocrine and immune systems in response to environment, circumstances, and the psychosocial factors that mediate these interactions (Caudell 1996).

> Interdisciplinary research efforts in 'psychoneuroimmunology' have provided compelling evidence of intimate connections between the brain and the immune system, as well as hints of the potential impact of such links for health and disease. (Bovbjerg and Valdimarsdottir 1998)

The traditional Western bio-medical model is grounded in the Cartesian and Newtonian paradigm, in which the mind, brain, and endocrine and immune systems are viewed principally as separate entities. Increasingly research is demonstrating the interrelatedness and dynamic interconnections between and within all systems providing a greater opportunity to address the whole of the human system and not just its separate parts (Ader *et al.* 1995; Bauer 1994).

Studies in PNI endeavour to explain how stress responses contribute to changes in the overall level of health, serving to draw a link between the degrees of health and illness. The focus of human-based PNI research has drawn on patient and associated client populations in clinical settings. Emphasis has been on symptom distress, life-threatening illness, bereavement, treatment side-effects, improving quality of life, strengthening immune system function, and enabling individuals to take a greater part in their own healing process through the use of relaxation, visualization, exercise, and nutrition (Ben-Eliyahu 1997; Berk *et al.* 2001; Caudell 1996; Kiecolt-Glaser and Glaser 1999; Schaub and Dossey 2000).

The precise way in which psychological and social factors influence and are influenced by the hormonal mediators of immune, neural, and endocrine functioning is still not completely understood. In essence, the evidence strongly indicates that the mind and body communicate with each other through a bi-directional flow of hormones, neuropeptides, and cytokines (Watkins 1997). Numerous neuroendocrine signals modulate immune response, with direct nerve-fibre connections stimulating communication between the central nervous system and primary and secondary lymphoid organs, and neurotransmitters exerting extensive regulatory control over immune responses. Cells of the immune system are capable of synthesizing neurohormones and nuerotransmitters directly.

In the presence of continual stress, whether in work, in home life, as a result of stressful life situations, or all of the above, there can be immune function impairment, notably immunosuppression, which particularly affects the function of lymphocyte and natural killer cells (Fillion 1996), with the ultimate consequence of illness or disease. It has been shown that states of depression, pain, and stressful events can impair immune system function (Zeller *et al.* 1996) and that there is a link between depression and cancer, particularly in the elderly who have been chronically depressed (Penninx *et al.* 1998).

The relevance of these findings to the study of stress in palliative care is reflected in the work of Brenninkmeyer *et al.* (2001) who differentiated burn-out from depression. Given that the clinical picture of depression seems to reflect a general sense of self-defeat, they hypothesized that individuals high in burn-out and low in superiority (how individuals see themselves in comparison to others) would experience depressive symptoms. Depressive symptomatology was highest among individuals high in burn-out who experienced a decline in superiority. They concluded that a reduced sense of superiority and a perceived loss of status were more characteristic of depressed individuals than of individuals who are burnt out.

The finding about depression is also relevant in view of the fact that depression and increased stress in palliative care staff were associated with the lack of participation in planning and decision making that may develop out of poor staff relationships (Cooper and Mitchell 1990; Alexander and MacLeod 1992; Hart *et al.* 1998). The conflict between hospice matrons and palliative care specialists in the UK regarding changing roles has also been reflected in stress in both groups (Finlay 1990; Graham *et al.* 1996). The conflict was hypothesized to derive in part from the lack of role clarity in the roles of consultants and senior nurses in palliative care because historically some charitably funded hospices were run by matrons (Graham *et al.* 1996).

Results from psycho-endocrine research has produced two notable findings. The first is that there are wide differences in endocrine responses that are influenced by the individual's perception of a stressful situation. Second, there is a wide range of hormones and neurotransmitters extended to cover an equally wide range of diseases (Watkins 1997). Data now intrinsically link psyche and soma, leading to the conclusion that immune modulation by psychosocial stressors can lead to changes in health (Bartlett 1998).

Pert (1997) illustrated the importance and critical involvement of emotions related to stressful events, stating that the accumulative effect and interpretation of any experience will stimulate a series of responses within the individual and that emotions become blocked which commonly arises from information overload. Pert suggests that when the mind–body networks are so overtaxed by sensory input, from unprocessed emotions and suppressed trauma, the individual becomes overwhelmed and bogged down. This process can lead to an unnatural state or order within the individual and may lead to disease-related stress. It is not a far step from this finding to conclude that if staff do not develop ways to deal with the stressors inherent in their work and professional lives they will be more vulnerable to illness. In the Netherlands, physician disability insurance premiums have risen 20 per cent to 30 per cent owing to an increasing incidence of burn-out and stress-related complaints (Ankone 1999).

Unless new memories or re-learning can take place there is a risk that the individual may not be able to move into more positive and proactive responses to stress. At a practical level, for example, if a caregiver has unresolved feelings about a previous death, then interactions with a currently dying person that remind one of the earlier experience may trigger a response that may not be relevant to the presenting situation.

If a staff member goes into a clinical situation with an openness to being compassionate and caring, it is more likely those actions will occur than if they go into the situation carrying unresolved issues from previous life experience, even unresolved issues from earlier in the day. Feelings of frustration and anger in either the caregiver or the client can rapidly spread to effect the other unless the caregiver is aware of their own feelings and how to deal with negative feelings that may be coming from the client.

Shaver (2002) has written that part of the experience of suffering is due to abandonment of the self, which occurs in childhood—these feelings emerge in the face of life-threatening illness. He notes that when the caregiver attempts to 'fix' the person, rather than validating their experience, the message being given is, 'the person that you are right now is not acceptable; let's substitute someone with whom we might both feel more comfortable'. Attempts to fix, therefore, may actually serve to exacerbate abandonment of self. A person dying of cancer who is angry at God can achieve more healing through acceptance and validation of their anger than through a theological debate. Psychospiritual healing requires a safe and supportive environment in which simply 'being in the presence of' carries tremendous healing potential (Shaver 2002).

Compassion fatigue

Concern has recently been expressed about the phenomenon of compassion stress or compassion fatigue. Compassion stress (also known as secondary traumatic stress (STS) (Figley 1995)) is said to result from closeness and exposure to repeated difficult illness experiences and deaths. Secondary traumatic stress is defined as 'the natural consequent behaviors and emotions resulting from knowing about a traumatizing event experienced by a significant other—the stress resulting from helping or wanting to help a traumatized or suffering person' (Figley 1995). Secondary traumatic stress disorder (STDS) is a more severe manifestation of STS and 'is a syndrome of symptoms nearly identical to PTSD (Post Traumatic Stress Disorder), except that exposure to knowledge about a traumatizing event experienced by a significant other is associated with the set of STSD symptoms, and PTSD symptoms are directly connected to the sufferer, the person experiencing the primary traumatic stress' (Figley 1995).

Garfield et al. (1995) writes of the compassion fatigue that exists amongst AIDS/HIV caregivers. He states that, in contrast to caregivers heading for burn-out who unconsciously begin to wall off more and more strong feelings associated with their work, those with compassion fatigue are able to monitor their decrease in empathy and feeling and remain emotionally accessible. However, they have greater and greater difficulty in processing their emotions, are anxiety ridden or distressed, and have images that intrude on their days and nights and painful memories that flood their world outside the caregiving arena . More research is needed in this area in palliative care to assess whether the phenomenon actually exists and if, with some of the coping mechanisms to be discussed below, it might be possible to alleviate the problem.

Management of self while caring for others

The heart has its reason which reason does not know. (French Proverb)

It is not uncommon for the heart to be used metaphorically in daily conversations, reflecting emotions. We are encouraged to 'take heart and not give up', to 'give it your whole heart', or to 'follow your heart'. Expressions of disappointment or loss of hope might include 'down-hearted', 'it was a heart-sink case', or 'feeling my heart was just not in it'. It is not surprising therefore to find the source of folklore is now implicated in the new evidence acknowledging the role of the heart in influencing and modulating the neurohormonal responses to stress and in the overall perception of well-being. Different emotional states, positive and negative, have been shown to affect the electrical rhythms generated by the heart. It is suggested that negative emotional states are immunosuppressive and that positive emotional states can enhance immunity (Watkins 1997).

The process of change and the rebalancing of life is central to health and well-being. Most of us seek recognition, inclusion, and acceptance and want to be viewed as 'normal'; when we encounter stress all of these facets can be altered. Emotional memory, learned behaviours, and social and professional expectations all contribute to our view of ourselves and that which gives our life meaning or creates what can become suffering. The effects of stress can lead to fragmentation between our thoughts, feelings, behaviours, and relationships and can challenge our very essence and what we expect of ourselves (Kearney 1996). Whenever there are expectations there is a risk of disappointment, which is a form of pain (Young-Eisendrath 2000). In caring for ourselves while we care for others it is important to have congruence between our thoughts, feelings, and actions aligned to our expectations. If these are aligned then we have a greater potential to stay awakened to the true nature of things and adjust our expectations accordingly. This does not mean that our personal standards have to be dropped, or compromised, rather more of using all of our intelligences, of thinking and feeling which when in balance helps us to maintain a reality on life, work, and ultimately health (Hayes 2000).

Remen (2000) speaks of the importance of meaning in life:

> Meaning is a form of strength. It has the power to transform experiences and even to open the most difficult of work to the dimension of joy and even gratitude. Meaning is the language of the soul.

She suggests that the concept of service underlies much of the work of the health professional:

> True service is not a relationship between an expert and a problem; it is far more genuine than that. It is a relationship between people who bring the full resources of their combined humanity to the table and share them generously.

She notes that many times when one helps one does not serve:

> When we help we become aware of our strength because we are using it. Others become aware of our strength as well and may feel diminished by it. But we do not serve with our strength; we serve with ourselves. We draw from all of our experiences … with parts of myself that embarrass me, parts of which I am ashamed. The wholeness in me serves the wholeness in others and the wholeness in life. Service is a relationship between equals.

Letting patients touch you requires opening to them and grieving when they die. Remen (1996) suggests that protecting ourselves from loss rather than grieving and healing our losses is one of the major causes of burn-out. People who do not care do not burn out:

> Only people who care can get into this place of numbness. We burn out not because we don't care but because we don't grieve. We burn out because we have allowed our hearts to become so filled with loss that we have no room left to care. (Remen 1996)

When we block off or deny the feelings of loss we have in this work using denial, rationalization, substitution, and avoidance, we numb the feeling of loss but at the same time we do not allow ourselves to find meaning or wisdom:

> Pain often marks the place where self-knowledge and growth can happen, much in the same way that fear does. (Remen 2000)

The way we approach caring for ourselves with be individually unique. Central to any steps we take to re-evaluate what we have to do to care for ourselves is the need to renew our attitude towards ourselves; only this way can the fragmentation be healed. The way to achieve self-care and to make changes that will enhance our lives can be best approached on an incremental basis. It is so often difficult to find the time to 'relax' and renew when by necessity or intention daily life is already very full and the thought of finding more time can be daunting. Whether one takes a pragmatic, problem-solving approach or a more expansive approach will be dependent on personal levels of energy, motivation, social support, and the ability to feel deserving of care.

It is important to understand those things that separate us from our instincts and feelings and lead us out of balance and harmony

> The place in which you find yourself isn't nearly as important as where you place your attention while you are there. (Paul and Collins 1992)

The following points are offered for your reflection.

1. Where are your efforts and energies predominately focused?

2. Is there a balance or a bias between your professional life and personal life?

3. Has there been a tendency to put off what you need to do for yourself in favour of others and their needs?

4. How do you reach your decisions over your priorities? What are the driving forces (within and outside of yourself) that influence these decisions?

5. Do you experience conflict within yourself over where you think or feel your attention needs to be? If so, how does this get resolved?

6. How often to find yourself 'doing good but feeling bad'?

7. What do you currently do to relieve stress? What do you find works best? What lasting effect does it provide?

8. What do you currently do for your own healing and renewal?

9. How easy is it for you to ask for and to receive support?

10. Do you achieve a balance between, work, rest, sleep, nutrition, and creativity?

11. What are the things that bring you meaning and purpose to your life?

Towards your own self-care and healing

Movement that fosters a commitment to improving the care of ourselves while caring for others requires a consistent concerted effort (Setch 2001). Individually we will have a natural or constitutional preference in the ways we approach our own healing needs. For some it will be through a process of reasoning, while for others it will arise out of emotions and feelings, and for others it will be through intuition or engagement with the body and senses (Benor 1996). The relevance of this lies in achieving the best self-care strategy, which will lead to enduring success.

Taking practical approaches to re-dressing the balance is often the first and most obvious helpful action towards making changes to improve our well-being and care of ourselves. With some reflection on the earlier questions take time to do the following.

1. Draw out your existing strategies and ways of prioritizing and coping with all aspects of your life.

2. Consider ways in which you would like to improve your life according to your goals. What improvements can be made immediately and which will need to take place over time.

There are now many books and programmes and a wide and diverse number of courses that teach and guide us towards the best techniques to enhance healthy approaches to life, self-care, and stress management; it is worth taking time to browse all resources to find what appeals to you and your life commitments.

When applying any method or strategies it is important to remember that no one method or technique is the exclusive answer; a combination of approaches with built-in flexibility is likely to bring about a richer response in the end. The salient point is to find what works for you and to give yourself the time for it. It is not uncommon to find that as health, balance, and insight are gained, the ways, means, and methods also change to reflect our progress.

The way forward as you seek to care for yourself

Ultimately the heads 'knows' but the heart 'understands'. (Childre and Howard 1999)

1. Stress management and self-care cannot be contained in isolation.

2. Endeavour to be proactive and not reactive in your stress management and lifestyle changes; making incremental, realistic changes over time is more effective than rushing or pushing to implement too many changes in one go.

3. Seek support and encouragement to avoid isolation.

4. Find ways to increase compassion for yourself in your daily life.

5. Foster a variety of experiences to sustain yourself while you seek to care for others.

6. Learn to tolerate the tension of struggle and conflict without collapsing into a judgment of 'this is good and this is bad'. Have realistic expectations of what can and cannot be achieved.

7. Engage in a variety of activities that can embrace all of your natural qualities and abilities.

Approaches

1. Utilize professional support systems, through clinical supervision and peer review.
2. Foster a habit of reflection both within the professional arena and your personal life.
3. Use methods and techniques that can assist the integration of the whole of you.

The scope of the chapter does not allow for an exhaustive list of techniques but highlights those that are relatively accessible. Emphasis should be on the development of effective responses in bringing about a state of relaxation that will help to reduce the effects of 'flight-and-fight' responses and might include some of the following groups of activities:

(1) relaxations that induce a deep muscle response, for example, progressive muscular, integrated relaxation methods such as autogenic training;

(2) relaxation through altered states, that is, self-hypnosis, guided imagery, and visualization;

(3) relaxation through touch, for example, massage, aromatherapy, reflexology; shiatsu, and therapeutic touch;

(4) techniques to assist in the release of difficult emotions and trauma including 'thought field therapy' and 'eye movement and desensitization programming';

(5) peer review and clinical supervision;

(6) regular exercise;

(7) taking time to reconnect with nature;

(8) attention to balanced nutrition and dietary supplements;

(9) reduction of stimulants, for example, caffeine, tobacco, and alcohol;

(10) maintaining a positive attitude and humour.

In addition to these approaches is the awareness of the need to respect our individual meanings and values for our lives and the honouring of that which we hold as precious or sacred within life. This can be achieved through meditation, contemplation, prayer, and the companionship with those people and events that enrich and nourish the process which brings us to a deeper inner connection to our true self.

Finally what is important is to find the balance through the choices you make towards your own needs. Unless we can achieve this for ourselves we are not likely to be able to achieve it for others.

References

Ader R, Cohen N, Felten DL (1995). Psychoneuroimmunology: interactions between the nervous system and immune system. *Lancet* **345**:99–103.

Alexander DA, MacLeod R (1992). Stress among palliative care matrons: a major problem for a minority group. *Palliative Med* **6**:111–24.

Alexander DA, Ritchie E (1990). 'Stressors' and difficulties in dealing with the terminal patient. *J Palliative Care* **6**:28–33.

Amenta MM (1984). Traits of hospice nurses compared with those who work in traditional settings. *J Clinl Psychol* **40:**414–19.

Amenta M (1995). Study reveals hospice nurses have a high degree of role satisfaction. *Fanfare* **IX:**18.

Ankone A (1999). Burnout among physicians almost doubled. *Medlisch Contact* **54:**494–7.

Bartlett D (1998). *Stress perspectives and processes*. Buckingham: Open University Press.

Bartol GM, Courts NF (2000). The physiology of bodymind healing. In: Dossey B, Keegan L, Guzzetta C (ed.). *Holistic nursing: a handbook for practice*. Aspen: Maryland.

Bauer SM (1994). Psychoneuroimmunology and cancer: an integrated view. *J Adv Nursing* **19:**114–20.

Beck-Friis B, Strang P, Sjödén P-O (1993). Caring for severely ill cancer patients: a comparison of working conditions in hospital-based home care and in hospital. *Support Care Cancer* **1:**145–51.

Bené B, Foxall MJ (1991). Death anxiety and job stress in hospice and medical-surgical nurses. *Hospice J* **7:**25–41.

Ben-Eliyahu S, Page GG, Yirmiya R, Shakhar G (1997). Evidence that stress and surgical interventions promote tumor developement by suppressing natural killer cells. *Int J Cancer* **80:**880–8.

Benor R (1996). A holistic view to managing stress. In Fisher RA, McDaid P (eds.). *Palliative Day Care*. London: Arnold.

Berk LS, Felten DL, Tan SA, Bittman BB (2001). Modulation of neuroimmune parameters during the eustress of humor-associated mirthful laughter. *Altern Ther* **7:**62–76.

Bovbjerg DH, Valdimarsdottir HB (1998). Psychoneuroimmunology: implications for psycho-oncology. In: JC Holland (ed.). *Psycho-Oncology*. New York: Oxford University Press. pp. 125–43.

Bowsher JE, Keep D (1995). Toward an understanding of three control constructs: personal control, self-efficacy and hardiness. *Iss Ment Health Nursing* **16:**33–50.

Bram PJ, Katz LF (1989). A study of burnout in nurses working in hospice and hospital oncology settings. *Oncol Nursing Forum* **16:**555–60.

Brenninkmeyer V, Van Yperen NW, Buunk BP (2001). Burnout and depression are not identical twins: is devline of superiority a distinguishing feature? *Personality Individ Diff* **30:**873–80.

Byock I (1998). Hospice and palliative care: a parting of the ways or a path to the future? *J Palliative Med* **1:**165–76.

Cassels D (1993). Tarnished images. Fall. Survey 1993: *The medical post national survey of Canadian doctors*. Toronto: Maclean Hunter.

Caudell KA (1996). Psychoneuroimmunology and innovative behavioural interventions in patients with Leukemia. *Oncol Nursing Forum* **23:**493–502.

Childre D, Martin H (1999). *The heartmarth solution. Proven techniques for developing emotional intelligence*. London: Piatkus.

Cho C, Cassidy DF (1994). Parallel processes for workers and their clients in chronic bereavement resulting from HIV. *Death Stud* **8:**273–92.

Cooper CL, Mitchell S (1990). Nursing the critically ill and dying. *Hum Relations* **43:**297–311.

Cooper CL, Rout U, Faragher B (1989). Mental health, job satisfaction, and job stress among general practitioners. *BMJ* **298:**366–70.

Copp G, Dunn V (1993). Frequent and difficult problems perceived by nurses caring for the dying in community, hospice and acute care settings. *Palliative Med* **7**:19–25.

Coyle N (1997). Focus on the nurse: ethical dilemmas with highly symptomatic patients dying at home. *Hospice J* **12**:33–41.

Deckard G, Meterko M, Field D (1994). Physician burnout: an examination of personal, professional, and organizational relationships. *Med Care* **32**:745–54.

D'Shano J (1996). Spiritual issues for patients and caregivers. In: Management of terminal illness: an update; 17–21 July. Ann Arbor, Michigan: International Hospice Institute.

Emerson J (1986). *Suffering: its meaning and ministry.* Nashville, Tennesee: Abingdon Press.

Figley CR (1995). Compassion fatigue as a secondary traumatic stress disorder: an overview. In: Figley CR (ed.). *Compassion fatigue.* New York: Brunner/Mazel. pp. 1–20.

Fillion L, Lemyre L, Manderville R, Piche R (1996). Cognitive apprasial, stress state, and cellular immunity response before and after diagnosis of breast tumor. *Int J Rehabilitation Health* **2**:169–87.

Finlay IG (1990). Sources of stress in hospice medical directors and matrons. *Palliative Med* **4**:5–9.

Fox M (1999). *Sins of the spirit, blessings of the flesh: lessons in transforming evil in soul and society.* New York: Three Rivers Press.

Franssén A (1997). *Omsorg i tanke og handling* [in Swedish, English summary]. Lund: Arkiv Förlag.

Garfield C, Spring C, Ober D (1995). *Sometimes my heart goes numb: love and caring in a time of AIDS.* San Fransisco: Jossey-Bass.

Graham J, Ramirez AJ, Cull A, Gregory WM, Finlay I, Hoy A *et al.* (1996). Job stress and satisfaction among palliative physicians: a CRC/ICRF study. *Palliative Med* **10**:185–94.

Gregory D, Russell CK (1999). *Cancer stories: on life and suffering.* Montreal: McGill-Queen's University Press.

Haigh C (2002). Using chaos theory: the implications for nursing. *J AdvNursing* **37**:462–9.

Hansen HP (1995). *I grænsefladen mellem liv og død* [in Danish]. Copenhagen: Gyldendals Boghandel.

Hart G, Yates P, Clinton M, Windsor C (1998). Mediating conflict and control: practice challenges for nurses working in palliative care. *Int J Nursing Stud* **35**:252–8.

Hayes RP (2000). A Buddha and his cousin. In: Young-Eisendrath P and Miller M (ed.). *The psychology of mature spirituality.* London: Routledge.

Heim E (1991). Job stressors and coping in health professions. *Psychother Psychosomat* **55**:90–9.

James N (1989). Emotional labour: skill and work in the social regulation of feelings. *Sociol Rev* **37**:15–42.

Kash K.M, Holland JC, Breitbart W, Brenson S, Dougherty J, Ouellette-Kobasa S (2000). Stress and burnout in oncology. *Oncology* **14**:1621–29.

Kearney M (1996). *Mortally wounded—stories of soul pain, death and healing.* Dublin: Marino Books.

Kiecolt-Glaser JK, Glaser R (1999). Psychoneuroimmunology and cancer: fact or fiction. *Eur J Cancer* **35**:1603–7.

Kobasa SC (1979). Stressful life events, personality and health: an inquiry into hardiness. *J Personality Soc Psychol* **37**:1–11.

Kobasa SC, Maddi SR, Courington S (1982). Hardiness and health: a prospective study. *J Personality Soc Psychol* **42**:168–77.

Kuuppelomäki M. and Lauri S (1998). Ethical dilemmas in the care of patients with incurable cancer. *Nursing Ethics* **5**:283–93.

Little D (1989). Human suffering in comparative perspective. In: Taylor RL, Watson J (ed.). *They shall not hurt: human suffering and human caring*. Boulder, Colorado: Colorado Associated University Press.

Longaker C (1997). Facing death and finding hope: a guide to the emotional and spiritual care of the dying. New York: Doubleday.

McMurray JE, Linzer M, Konrad TR, Douglas J, Shugerman R, Nelson K (for the SGIM Career Satisfaction Study Group) (2000). The work lives of women physicians: results from the physician work life study. *J Gen Intern Med* **15**:372–80.

Maslach C, Jackson SE (1982). Burnout in health professions: a social psychological analysis. In: Sanders GS, Suls J (ed.) *Social psychology of health and illness*. London: Erlbaum.

Maslach C, Jackson SE (1986). *Maslach burnout inventory manual*. Palo Alto: Consulting Psychologists Press.

Mount BM (1986). Dealing with our losses. *J Clin Oncol* **4**:1127–34.

Nowack KM (1990). Initial development of an inventory to assess stress and health risk. *Am J Health Promotion* **4**:173–80.

Papadatou D (2000). A proposed model of health professionals' grieving process. *Omega* **41**:59–77.

Papadatou D, Anagnostopoulos F, Monos D (1994). Factors contributing to the development of burnout in oncology nursing. *BrJ Med Psychol* **67**:187–99.

Paul SC, Collins GM (1992). *Inneractions: visions to bring your inner and outer worlds into harmony*. San Fransisco: Harper.

Payne N (2001). Occupational stressors and coping as determinants of burnout in female hospice nurses. *J Adv Nursing* **33**:396–405.

Penninx BW, Guralnik JM, Pahor M, Ferrucci L, Cerhan JR, Wallace RB *et al.* (1998). Chronically depressed mood and cancer risk in older persons. *J Nat Cancer Inst* **90**:1888–93.

Pert C (1997). *Molecules of Emotion*. UK: Simon and Schuster.

Ramirez AJ, Graham J, Richards MA, Cull A, Gregory WM, Leaning MS *et al.* (1995). Burnout and psychiatric disorder among cancer clinicians. *Br J Cancer* **71**:1263–9.

Rasmussen BH, Sandman P-O (2000). Nurses' work in a hospice and in an oncological unit in Sweden. *Hospice J* **15**:53–75.

Remen RN (1996). *Kitchen table wisdom*. New York: Riverhead Books.

Remen RN (2000). *My grandfather's blessings*. New York: Riverhead Books.

Robbins RA (1991). Death anxiety, death competency and self-actualization in hospice volunteers. *Hospice J* **7**:29–35.

Schaub BG, Dossey BM (2000). Imagery: awakening the inner healer. In: Dossey BM, Keegan L, Guzzetta CE (ed.). *Holistic nursing: a handbook for practice*. Maryland: Aspen.

Setch F (2001). Looking after yourself. In: Kinghorn S, Gamlin R (ed.). *Palliative nursing: bringing comfort and hope*. London: Bailliere and Tindall.

Shapiro DH Jr, Schwartz CE, Astin JA (1996). Controlling ourselves, controllong our world: psychology's role in understanding positive and negative consequences of seeking and gaining control. *Am Psychol* **51**:1213–30.

Sharpley CF, Dua JK, Reynolds R, Acosta A (1995). The direct and relative efficacy of cognitive hardiness, type A behaviour pattern, coping behaviour and social support as predictors of stress and ill-health. *ScandJ Behav Ther* **24**:15–29.

Shaver WA (2002). Suffering and the role of abandonment of self. *J Hospice Palliative Nursing* **4:**46–53.

Simoni PS, Paterson JJ (1997). Hardiness, coping, and burnout in the nursing workplace. *J Profess Nursing* **13:**178–85.

Stein J (ed.-in-Chief), Urdang L (Managing ed.) (1967). *The Random House dictionary of the English language.* Unabridged edn. New York: Random House.

Taylor EJ, Highfield MF, Amenta M (1999). Predictors of oncology and hospice nurses' spiritual care perspectives and practices. *Appl Nursing Res* **12:**30–7.

Trygstad L (1986). Professional friends: the inclusion of the personal into the professional. *Cancer Nursing* **9:**326–32.

Vachon MLS (1987). *Occupational stress in the care of the critically ill, the dying and the bereaved.* New York: Hemisphere Press.

Vachon MLS (1995). Staff stress in palliative/hospice care: a review. *Palliative Med* **9:**91–122.

Vachon MLS (2000). Burnout and symptoms of stress in staff working in palliative care. In: Chochinov HM, Breitbart W (ed.). *Handbook of psychiatry in palliative medicine.* New York: Oxford University Press. pp. 303–19.

Vachon MLS (2001). The nurse's role: the world of palliative care nursing. In: Ferrell B, Coyle N (ed.). *The Oxford textbook of palliative nursing.* New York: Oxford University Press. pp. 647–62.

Watkins A (1997). Mind–body pathways. In: Watkins A (ed.). *Mind–body medicine: a clinician's guide to psychoneuroimmunology.* Edinburgh: Churchill Livingstone.

Watson J (1989). Human caring and suffering: a subjective model for health sciences. In: Taylor RL, Watson J (ed.). *They shall not hurt: human suffering and human caring.* Boulder, Colorado: Colorado Associated University Press. pp. 125–35.

Young-Eisendrath P (2000). Psychotherapy as ordinary transcendence: the unspeakable and the unspoken. In: Young-Eisendrath P, Miller M (ed.). *The psychology of mature spirituality.* London: Routledge.

Zeller J, McCain N.J, Swanson B (1996). Psychoneuroimmunology: an emerging framework for nursing research. *J Adv Nursing* **23:**657–64.

Zerwekh J (1993). Transcending life:the practice wisdom of nursing hospice experts. *Am J Hospice Palliative Care* **5:**26–31.

Chapter 12

Psychosocial care—the future

Mari Lloyd-Williams

Introduction

This book has looked at the issues of providing psychosocial care within palliative care, but what of the future? What sort of care do we envisage providing for our patients? How can we ensure that each patient receives full and optimum psychosocial care in the same way as they received full and optimum medical treatment? What are the areas we need to develop in psychosocial care in order to provide better care for the future? This chapter will try to address these questions.

What do patients want?

Breaking bad news is challenging. What we say and what the patient may hear or understand may be very different, leading to misunderstanding and not infrequently bitterness and resentment against the bearer of the bad news. Whilst many patients may have an inkling that all is not well, the desire to hear good news can also prevent information from being heard and assimilated. Giving bad news in whatever setting is never easy for the bearer—nor should it be, but certain steps can help a diagnosis or prognosis to be given in a means whereby patients understand what is being said and feel supported.

When discussing psychological care it is important to remember that it is the quality of the relationships between patients and their professional carers that promotes the disclosure of psychosocial information—patients feel able to share their deepest distresses when they sense a caring approach (Doyle 1996).

Historically, there has been a perception that distressing information was best kept hidden from patients but several studies have shown that the vast majority of patients want specific information regarding their diagnosis and prognosis (Jenkins *et al.* 2001; McIllmurray *et al.* 2001). Despite many innovations in both medical and nursing curricula with regard to communication skills, poor communication of information or the mode that the communication was conveyed comprise the single largest cause for complaints by patients about their care. Effective communication skills are the key to providing effective cancer and palliative care (Fallowfield and Jenkins 1999). A paper by Rogers *et al.* (2000) described how patients perceived that all the services were excellent but it was the human element that caused things to go wrong and caused the patients and their families pain and distress (Mager and Andrykowski 2002). The ability to learn communication skills has been detailed in Chapter 2 of this book. Training in communication skills can improve professional skills (Fallowfield and Jenkins 2002) and additionally can alter beliefs and attitude (Jenkins and Fallowfield 2002). However improved communication skills do not always improve the ability of medical and nursing staff to detect psychosocial distress in their patients (Ford *et al.* 1994; Fallowfield *et al.* 2001). Whilst research into communication skills training is important, it is vital that skills are transferred into practice and that patients benefit. A recent much publicized book has criticized health professionals for their insensitive approach to a young patient with a terminal illness (Clark 2002). More research is needed on healthcare staff behaviour and why professionals who know the theory of good communication are unable to translate this into practice.

Provision of psychosocial care

For many patients, the presence of a caring, empathic professional who is able to give honest information sensitively will be adequate and appropriate. However, a significant number of patients have complex psychological and psychiatric needs either due to long-standing difficulties or as a result of their advanced malignant disease. The need for professionals with specific skills in psychosocial care in addition to those members of nursing and medical staff with generic skills has been identified for some time but the independent nature of many palliative care units and teams means that there are few standardized procedures for management of patients with specific needs. Seale (1989), when discussing psychosocial care, concluded that information was difficult to obtain and that there appeared to be a wide variation in the care available and offered to patients. The National Council for Hospices and Specialist Palliative Care Services (NCHSPCS) (an umbrella organization of palliative care representing professionals from different disciplines involved with care of the terminally ill patient) set up a working party to look more closely at the issues of psychosocial care and its provision. They published an occasional paper (National Council for Hospices and Specialist Palliative Care Services 1997), which amongst other statements defined psychosocial skills.

These skills were specified at three levels:

(1) level one—skills which are general communication skills desirable for all caregiving staff and volunteers;

(2) level two—skills including excellent interpersonal and communication skills which are appropriate to staff members with an extensive first-line role in palliative care, for example, clinical nurse specialists in palliative care;

(3) level three—skills which are required by a specialist in psychosocial care.

The paper further states that

> Central to the application of these skills is the ability of all staff to recognise when they have reached the ceiling of their skills, or the situation has become too complex, and to be able to refer appropriately.

Specialists in psychosocial care are specified as family therapists and social workers, chaplains and spiritual advisers, psychologists, and psychiatrists. Staff therefore need to be aware of the patients who may benefit from referral to another professional either from within the team itself, or a designated person who is known to the team. It is often relatively straightforward to know when a patient requires intervention from a social worker to help them sort out future care for a dependent relative or financial support but it may be more difficult to know when intervention from a psychologist or psychiatrist may be required. The provision of psychosocial care within palliative care in the UK appears to be *ad hoc* unlike in the USA where services are well developed and integrated. A survey published of 166 hospices in the UK in 1999 (Lloyd-Williams *et al.* 1999) found that whilst all units had access to a chaplain and the majority social workers (75 per cent), less than 10 per cent of units had regular support from psychologists or psychiatrists. Additionally the manpower shortage of both these professions and the length of time taken for a patient to be seen meant that the services were rarely utilized (Guthrie 1998). The regular provision of psychiatry or psychology is welcomed by units and influences both appropriate referrals and treatment decisions (Mitchell 1998; Montgomery 1999). A lack of adequate liaison psychiatry and psychology services is identified as a limiting factor in providing adequate psychosocial care for patients by the majority of palliative care consultants (Lawrie and Lloyd-Williams in press).

Many units and teams are unable to provide statistics on the numbers of patients or relatives seen by psychosocial services (Lloyd-Williams *et al.* 1999) again suggesting that these may operate in an *ad hoc* fashion and many services listed art therapists, volunteer befrienders, counsellors, and complementary therapists as being members of their psychosocial team. All of these people would see themselves and be seen by others as providing psychosocial care and of being 'companions' for patients with a terminal illness (Thompson *et al.* 2001). The mechanisms for supervision for such services within palliative care is poor and there is little information as to whether patients with more complex needs are referred onto other services.

Walker *et al.*, in Chapter 4 of this book, have described and proposed models of service delivery; such services frequently include complementary therapies for example, which although have not been specifically mentioned in this book are considered an essential component of psychosocial care. All such interventions require careful evaluation to ensure that patients are offered appropriate support at the appropriate time and that all interventions have been evaluated for effectiveness. The old adage that not everything that is important can be measured may well come to mind but it is essential that psychosocial care continues to explore by rigorous means which interventions are effective.

Complex psychosocial needs

The hierarchy of psychosocial care has been identified by the NCHSPCS and Chapter 4 has proposed models as to how effective and appropriate psychosocial care can be delivered. The need for assessment is paramount. Much work has been carried out on developing tools for the assessment of psychosocial care (Wright *et al.* 2001) and others have looked at whether psychosocial distress can be predicted or is associated with cancer site (Zabora *et al.* 2001; Ciarmella and Poli 2001; Kurtz *et al.* 2002).

Assessment tools such as Intermed (Mazzocato *et al.* 2000) have aimed to develop a method whereby psychosocial information is collected routinely at any assessment. All these studies and others conclude that those professionals closest to the patients, typically nursing and medical staff, need to be aware when patients require more than 'blanket' psychosocial support and need further referral. If we consider depression as an example, two recent studies (Lloyd-Williams and Payne in press*a*; Lloyd-Williams and Payne in press*b*) have looked at how clinical nurse specialists, who frequently have a very close relationship with advanced cancer patients, assess and manage depression in their patients. A quantitative study found that 79 per cent of all clinical nurse specialists believed that their skills were poor in the assessment of depression in palliative care patients and 92 per cent perceived that they required further training. These highly qualified and skilled nurses were unsure of which symptoms of depression were significant in palliative care patients and additionally were frequently isolated and had no mechanism for referral of further assessment. The qualitative study explored specialist nurses' views on depression in palliative care and found that many nurses found it difficult to discuss depression with their patients and tended to focus on physical symptoms. The lack of training in identifying psychological and psychiatric symptoms was a source of concern to the nurses themselves as were the difficulties they also encountered in trying to persuade medical staff that patients required further assessment or anti-depressant medication. There is also a need for randomized controlled trials to determine which interventions are most appropriate and effective for palliative care patients (Ly *et al.* 2002).

The future of psychosocial care

The need for palliative care to be extended to all patient groups with end-stage disease and not only cancer has been identified (National Council for Hospice and Specialist Palliative Care 1998). Such patients may also have many complex psychosocial needs in addition to symptom-control needs. Many of these patients will have lived with a chronic illness for some time; the rates of psychological distress and depression is high in these patient groups (McCarthy *et al.* 1996) but frequently is not addressed. Patients with existing complex psychosocial needs also develop terminal illness (National Council for Hospices and Specialist Palliative Care Services 2000) and require access to palliative care services. It is important that links with their existing social and psychological care services are kept in order for palliative care teams to be able to offer ongoing care. The focus in palliative care in recent years has been to ensure that patients are offered symptom control from point of need, which in some patients may be diagnosis, and that this support is ongoing. In the early days of the clinical nurse specialist, nurses were frequently present when patients were informed that treatment was palliative or when patients were being told that treatment would be discontinued. Specialist nurses continued to provide ongoing support and assessment for such patients. As palliative care teams become more acutely focused and resources stretched, the emphasis on the control of physical symptoms has tended to take priority. Specialist nurses are increasingly being used as an acute resource and palliative care consultants rarely have the opportunity to develop their own caseload, their role being predominantly to troubleshoot acute physical symptoms. Providers of psychosocial care and palliative care need to ensure wider access to services and that all professionals are able to understand and differentiate between those patients who need 'companioning' (that is, all patients) and those patients who have more complex psychosocial needs and require referral to a more appropriate person. Whilst integration of services is essential, as is wider access across more disease areas, it is also important to acknowledge that the control of physical symptoms is only 25 per cent of our remit—the psychological, social, and spiritual aspects of palliative care are what have made palliative care a separate entity, and ensuring high quality research in these areas is a priority for the future.

References

Ciarmella A, Poli P (2001). Assessment of depression among cancer patients: the role of pain, cancer type and treatment. *Psycho-oncology* **10:**156–65.

Clark R (2002). *A long walk home.* Oxford: Radcliffe Press.

Dogle D (1996). Education in palliative medicine. *Palliative Medicine* **10:**91–92.

Fallowfield L, Jenkins V (1999). Effective communication skills are the key to good cancer care. *Eur J Cancer* **35:**1592–7.

Fallowfield L, Jenkins V (2002). Efficacy of a cancer research UK communication skills training model for oncologists: a randomised controlled trial. *Lancet* **359:**650–6.

Fallowfield L, Ratcliffe D, Jenkins V, Saul J (2001). Psychiatric morbidity and its recognition by doctors in patients with cancer. *Br J Cancer* **84:**1011–15.

Ford S, Fallowfield L, Lewis S (1994). Can oncologists detect distress in their outpatients and how satisfied are they with their performance during bad news consultations? *Br J Cancer* **70:**767–770.

Guthrie E (1998). Development of liaison psychiatry. *Psychiat Bull* **22:**291–3.

Jenkins V, Fallowfield L, Saul J (2001). Information needs of patients with cancer: results from a large study of cancer centres. *BrJ Cancer* **5:**48–51.

Jenkins V, Fallowfield L (2002). Can communication skills training alter physicians' beliefs and behaviours in clinics? *J Clin Oncol* **20:**765–9.

Kurtz M, Kurtz J, Stommel M, Given C, Given B (2002). Predictors of depressive sympomatology of geriatric patients with lung cancer—a longitudinal analysis. *Psycho-oncology* **11:**12–22.

Lawrie I, Lloyd-Williams M (in press). How do palliative care physicians care for patients with depression?

Lloyd-Williams M, Friedman T, Rudd N (1999). A survey of psychosocial service provision within hospices. *Palliative Med* **13:**431–2.

Lloyd-Williams M, Payne S (in press*a*). Nurse specialist assessment and management of palliative care patients who are depressed—a study of perceptions and attitudes. *J Palliative Care.*

Lloyd-Williams M, Payne S (in press*b*). A qualitative study of the role of clinical nurse specialists in the assessment of depression in palliative care patients. *Palliative Med.*

Ly K, Chidgey J, Addington-Hall J, Hotopf M (2002). Depression in palliative care: a systematic review. *Palliative Med* **16:**279–84.

Mager W, Andrykowski M (2002). Communication in the cancer 'bad news' consultation: patient perceptions and psychological adjustment. *Psycho-oncology* **11**:35–46.

Mazzocato C, Stiefel F, de Jonge P, Levorato A, Ducret S, Huyse F (2000). Comprehensive assessment of patients in palliative care: a descriptive study utilising the Intermed. *J Pain Sympt Manage* **19**:83–90.

McCarthy M, Lay M, Addington-Hall J (1996). Dying form heart disease. *J Royal Coll Phys* **30**:325–8.

McIllmurray M, Thomas C, Francis B, Morris S, Soothill K, Al-hamad A (2001). The psychosocial needs of cancer patients:findings from an observational study. *Eur J Cancer Care* **10**:261–9.

Mitchell J (1998). Psychiatric involvement in an Edinburgh hospice. *Psychiat Bull* **22**:172–3.

Montgomery C (1999). Psycho-oncology: a coming of age. *Psychiat Bul* **23**:431–5.

National Council for Hospice and Specialist Palliative Care Services (1997). Feeling better—psychosocial care in specialist palliative care. Occasional Paper Number 13. London.

National Council for Hospices and Specialist Palliative Care Services (1998). Reaching out: specialist palliative care for adults with non-malignant disease. London.

National Council for Hospices and Specialist Palliative Care Services and Scottish Partnership Agency for Palliative and Cancer Care (2000). Positive partnerships—palliative care for adults with severe mental health problems. London.

Rogers A, Karslen S, Addington-Hall J (2000). All the services were excellent. It is when the human element comes in that things go wrong: dissatisfaction with hospital care in the last year of life. *J Adv Nursing* **31**:768–73.

Seale C (1989). What happens in hospices: a review of the research evidence. *Soc Sci Med* **28**:551–9.

Thompson M, Rose C, Wainwright W, Matter L, Scanlan M (2001). Activities of counsellors in a hospice/palliative care environment. *J Palliative Care* **17**:229–35.

Wright E, Selby P, Gould A, Cull A (2001). Detecting social problems in cancer care. *Psycho-oncology* **10**:242–50.

Zabora J, Brintzenhoefeszoc K, Curbow B, Hooker C, Piantadosi S (2001). The prevalence of psychological distress by cancer sites. *Psycho-oncology* **10**:19–28.

Index